DENTAL IMPLANTS: THE COMPLETE PATIENT'S GUIDE

George Ghidrai
MD

Contents

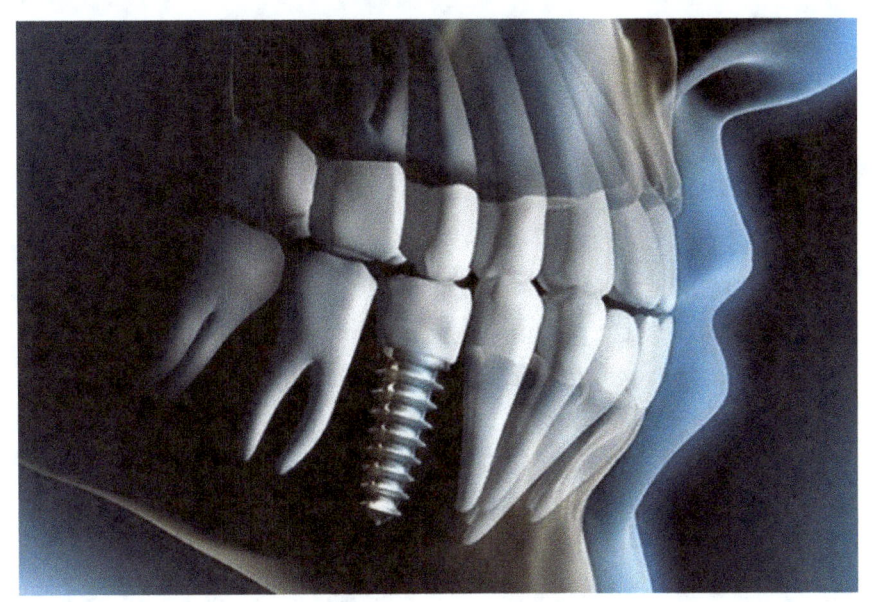

1. Introduction

◆◆◆

Today, dental implants are state-of-the-art tooth replacement systems and are now more common than ever before.

Losing a tooth, whether due to injury, decay, or age, can be a daunting experience. It affects not only your ability to eat, speak, and smile but also your overall quality of life. Dental implants can fix this problem in the most natural way, making your new teeth feel and work just like your real ones.

However, figuring out how to get dental implants can be confusing as it requires patients to navigate a maze of choices, from implant types and procedures to aftercare and maintenance.

Dental Implants: The Complete Patient's Guide is designed to help you understand all the important aspects of dental implants so you can make informed decisions about your dental health. It doesn't matter if you're just considering getting dental implants or want to know more about the process. This book can be your go-to resource for understanding the entire procedure.

We'll start with the basics of dental implants. You will learn what dental implants are, how they work, their main benefits, and their success rate. You will also discover when dental implants are strongly indicated, how much they cost, and why dental implant restorations are superior to traditional dental bridges.

We will also delve into the different types of dental implants and implant-supported restorations, discussing considerations like materials, structure, shapes, and sizes.

Understanding the dental implant procedure is essential, and we'll take you through each step, from your first meeting with the dentist to the care you'll need after the surgery.

We'll also explore the different treatment options, like replacing one tooth, several teeth, or even all your teeth with dental implants.

This guide goes beyond the clinical aspects of dental implants. It also covers key topics like oral health maintenance, hygiene, and long-term care, ensuring your investment in dental implants remains successful for years. We will address common concerns and questions, such as risks and complications and possible reasons for failure. We even have a chapter about Laboratory Stages and how implant restorations are constructed at the dental lab.

This book is written in an easy-to-understand language, and each topic is clearly illustrated; this allows anyone to walk through each stage of this guide and easily grasp the information they need.

Whether you're concerned about aesthetics, functionality, or overall health, *Dental Implants: The Complete Patient's Guide* is designed to inform, support, and guide you every step of the way.

One final important notice before we get started: you should not use this guide as a substitute for professional medical advice, diagnosis, or treatment. Always seek the advice of your dental implantologist with any questions you may have, and never disregard professional medical advice or delay in seeking it.

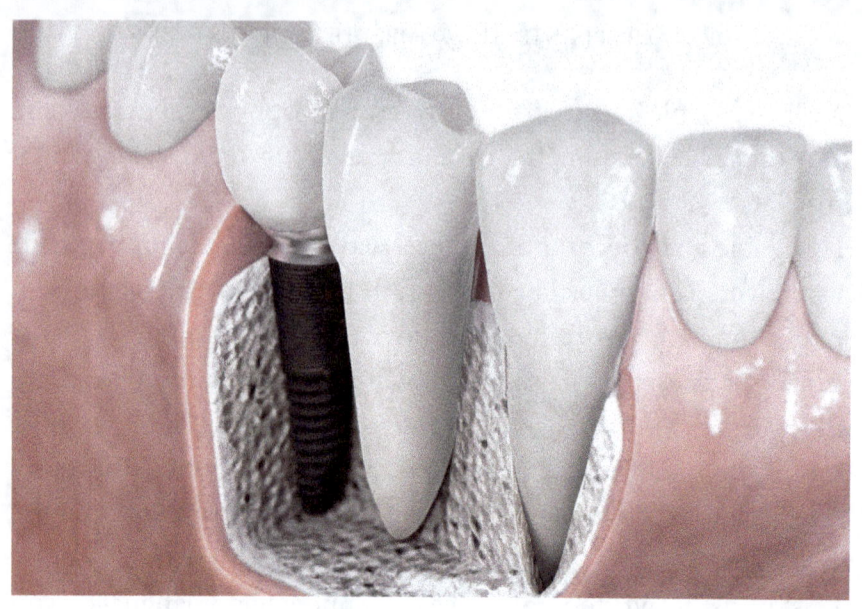

2. General Considerations

♦♦♦

2.1 What Are Dental Implants?

Dental implants are metal devices surgically inserted into the jawbone to replace one or more missing teeth. Dental implants typically support a dental prosthesis such as a crown, bridge, or removable dentures, but sometimes, they may act as an orthodontic anchor (to align and straighten teeth).

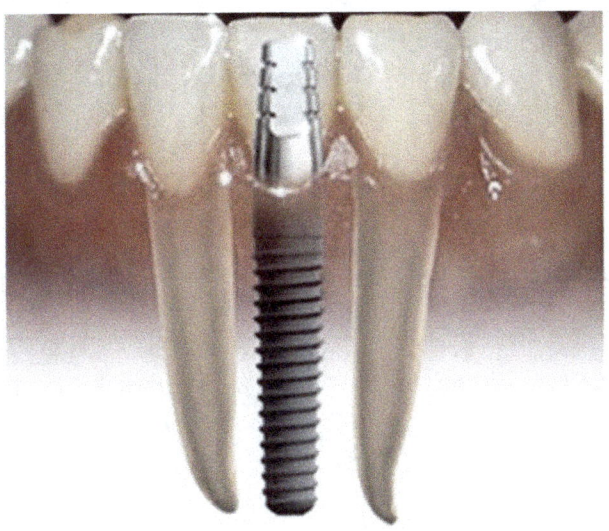

First, a surgical procedure is required to place the dental implant inside the jawbone. The basis for modern dental implants is a biological process called *osseointegration*, where materials such as titanium form an intimate bond to the bone. Osseointegration requires a variable amount of healing time (usually 3 to 6 months).

After the healing time, an abutment is attached to the implant. The abutment will hold the dental prosthesis (crown, bridge, removable denture).

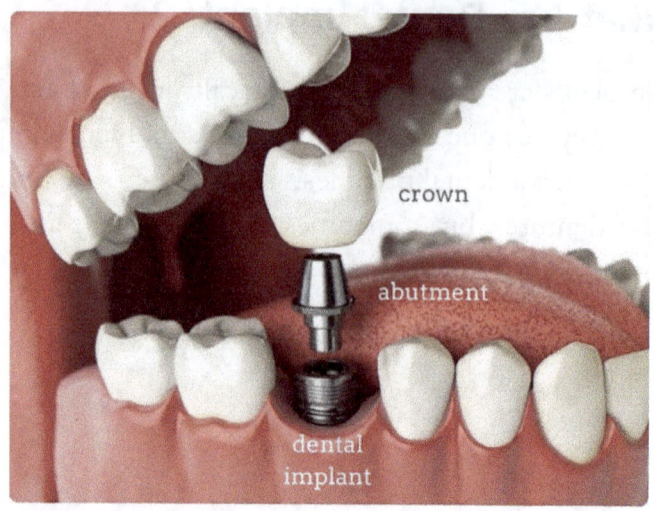

Implantology

Dental implantology is a set of surgical techniques aiming at the functional rehabilitation of a patient affected by total or partial edentulism by using dental implants.

What is *Edentulism*?

> **• Edentulism is a medical condition characterized by the absence of one or more teeth. This medical condition is caused by loss of teeth.**

Dental implantology is a relatively new dental subspecialty (the primary specialty is oral and maxillofacial surgery).
In later years, because of the ever-increasing demand for dental implants, implantology experienced a spectacular development:

☐ new surgical techniques appeared,

☐ new materials were developed,

☐ new rehabilitation methods were devised,

all aimed at increasing the quality and success rate of dental implants.

For these reasons, techniques and solutions differ from one practitioner to another and from one region or country to another.

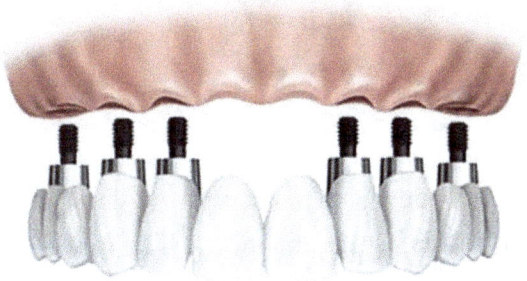

implant-supported dental bridge

Why is it so important to replace missing teeth?

Following teeth loss, several toothless spaces appear inside the oral cavity. These are called edentulous spaces or toothless gaps.

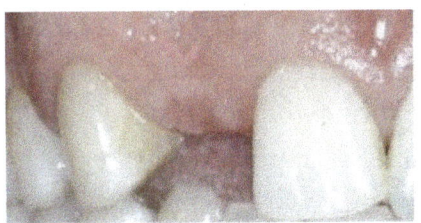 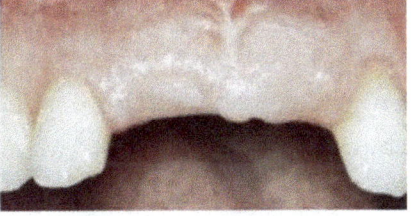

single tooth gap   *several teeth gap*

If toothless gaps are not rehabilitated in time (with a dental restoration), irreversible changes may occur around these areas, adversely affecting oral health.

Let's review some of the changes that may occur following a tooth extraction.

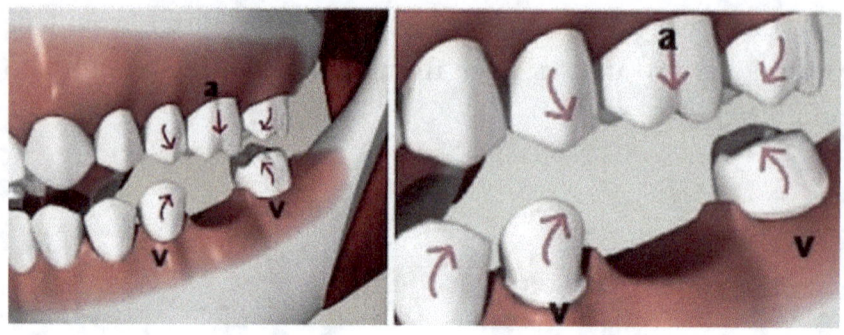

- **Opposite teeth**, marked with *a*, migrate towards the extraction site (overeruption). The process occurs until the tooth reaches the opposite gum (called the edentulous ridge) or another obstacle located on the path.
- **Adjacent teeth**, marked with *v*, lean toward the edentulous space in an attempt "to close the gap."

Teeth migration stops when the toothless gap is restored with a dental prosthesis.

Teeth migration can disrupt the most important oral processes: mastication, aesthetics, and phonation. Moreover, migrated teeth can suffer from periodontal diseases or cavities.

The space required for manufacturing the reconstruction will gradually diminish and eventually disappear altogether. Any prosthesis, including implant-supported dentures, needs adequate room for artificial teeth to be shaped appropriately.

If the required space diminishes because of teeth migration, preliminary operations (most often complicated and expensive) are needed before the design of the prosthetic restoration can actually begin.

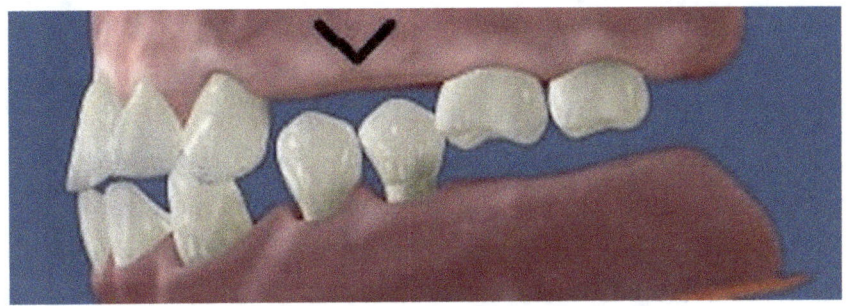

a case of over-eruption that leads to the
vertical shrinkage of the toothless gap

Conclusion

!!! After teeth extractions, it is essential to restore the toothless gaps as soon as possible. As you will see in this chapter, dental implants offer superior therapeutic solutions compared to traditional restorations (such as dental bridges or removable dentures supported by natural teeth).

2.2 Dental Implants. Role, Benefits, Success Rate

What are dental implants' primary purposes?

Many patients may wonder why they should choose dental implants (which are more expensive) over traditional dental restorations supported by natural teeth.

The great advantage of a dental implant is that it replaces the missing tooth in the most natural way possible. Dental implants "fuse" with the bone thanks to the biological process called osseointegration (we will discuss more about osseointegration later in this book).

Thanks to this process, implant-supported prostheses offer a variety of advantages compared to conventional restorations.

The main objective of any dental implant restoration is properly replacing the missing teeth.

Teeth have three functions: Chewing, Aesthetics, and Pronunciation. The main goal of any dental restoration is to restore these functions as close as possible to natural teeth.

Let's compare implant restorations to traditional restoration in rehabilitating teeth's main functions:

• Mastication or chewing process

Mastication is a fundamental dental process. When a dental prosthesis is designed, restoring this process as closely as possible to natural teeth is essential. The patient will quickly accommodate the new restoration when this goal is achieved.

For example, when an implant-supported denture is manufactured, the chewing forces are passed to the surrounding bone, just *like natural teeth* (see image). Consequently, chewing comfort is excellent because dental implants function remarkably like natural teeth.

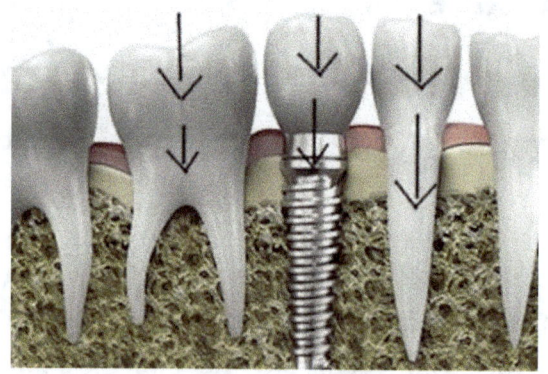

chewing forces in case of a dental implant

By contrast, when a traditional denture is designed, some chewing forces are passed to the underneath gums, as dentures usually rest exclusively on the gums.

Because the gum tissues are not used to withstand excessive pressure, it will take longer to get used to traditional removable dentures.

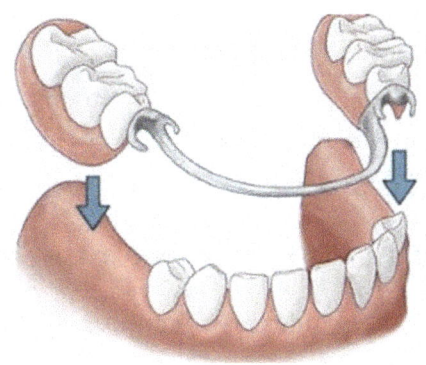

chewing forces in case of removable dentures

• Aesthetics

Restoring aesthetics is, for many patients, the most important goal. The general aesthetic of an implant-supported reconstruction is **excellent**. A dental implant restores a lost tooth to look, feel, fit, and function almost like a natural tooth.

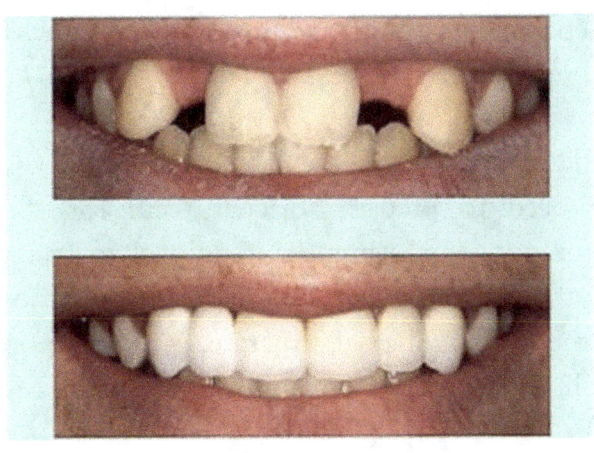

restoring aesthetics with
two implant-supported crowns

• *Phonation or pronunciation*

Standard speech can be disrupted when the front upper teeth (particularly incisors) are missing. It is well known that these teeth are essential in pronouncing some consonants.

Adjusting to traditional removable dentures can mean struggling to pronounce everyday words until mouth tissues adapt to the new situation (which can take several weeks); not so with dental implants, which function almost like natural teeth.

What are dental implants' essential advantages?

As we said, the most significant advantage of dental implants is how they replace missing teeth. Implants "fuse" with the bone thanks to the biological process called osseointegration, and, as a result, they function like natural teeth.

Thanks to this process, implant-supported prostheses offer a variety of advantages compared to conventional restorations.

- Dental implants reduce the load on the remaining oral structures (teeth, gums, jawbone) by offering independent support and retention to crowns, bridges, and removable dentures.

- Dental implants preserve natural tooth tissue by avoiding the need to prepare adjacent teeth for conventional restorations (for example, a traditional dental bridge).
  Tooth preparation involves permanently removing parts of the tooth's original structure, including portions that might still be healthy and structurally sound.

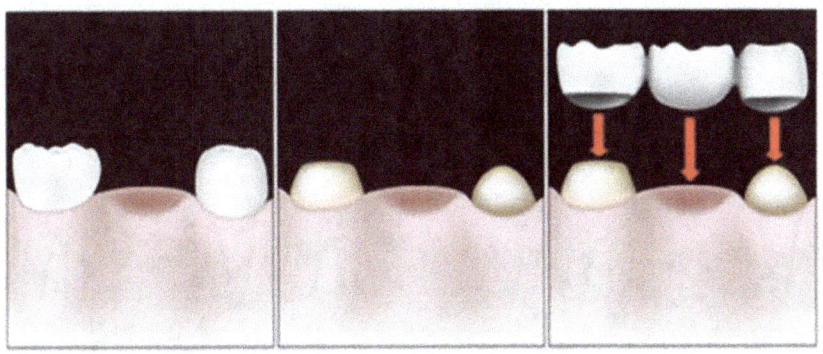

single tooth gap: if a traditional dental bridge is designed, the preparation of the adjacent teeth is required

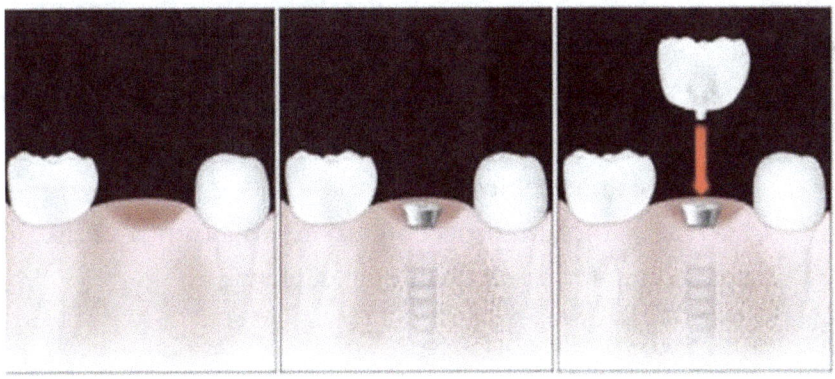

single tooth gap: if an implant-supported crown is manufactured, the adjacent teeth remain untouched

- Dental implants will preserve bone and significantly reduce bone resorption and deterioration. Bone resorption always results in loss of jawbone height or width.
- Implant-supported dentures allow you to chew the food better and speak more clearly. Studies have shown that these prostheses improve chewing efficiency and speaking compared to complete dentures (also known as full dentures).

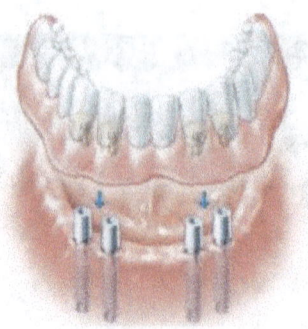
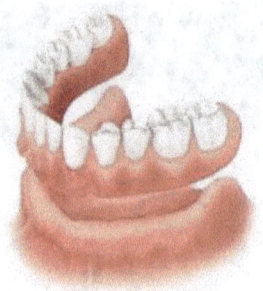

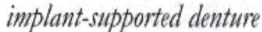

implant-supported denture   *complete denture*

What are the main drawbacks?

Dental implants have few drawbacks if there are no general or local contraindications (we will discuss these later).

- A surgical procedure for implant placement and a healing period is necessary before the definitive prosthesis is completed.
- Dental implant procedures may entail an increase in cost compared to conventional dentistry.

Success rate

Because of constant developments in the field of implantology, the success rate of dental implants has continually risen.

In the presence of healthy tissues, a well-integrated implant with appropriate biomechanical loads can have long-term success rates of 93 to 98 percent for the fixture and 10 to 15 years lifespan for the prosthetic teeth.

Several factors can influence the success rate of dental implants:

- **The quality and quantity of the available bone**: Implants placed in thicker, stronger bone have a higher success rate. Sometimes, adjunctive surgical procedures are performed to increase the height or width of the alveolar bone.

14

We will discuss adjunctive surgical procedures in a later chapter.

• **Case complexity**: Young and healthy patients with relatively simple restorations (e.g., single tooth missing) have a higher success rate.

• **Care And Maintenance**: Taking good care of dental implants is vital for long-term success. You will learn how to take care of your implants later in this book.

• **Quality of the medical practitioner**: It goes without saying that experienced implant specialists have a higher success rate.

2.3 Indications, Contraindications

When are dental implants strongly indicated?

Dental implants can successfully restore all forms of Edentulism: from Partial Edentulism, when one or more teeth are missing, to Complete Edentulism, when all teeth from a dental arch are missing.

If there are no general or local contraindications, implant-supported restorations are the *method of choice* in restoring all types of toothless gaps.

In certain clinical situations, dental implants are strongly recommended over traditional restorations:

• Single unit toothless gap with healthy adjacent teeth

When a single tooth is missing, an implant-supported crown will preserve the adjacent natural teeth by avoiding the need to prepare them.

If the toothless gap is restored with a traditional *dental bridge*, both adjacent teeth will have to be prepared. This operation

15

involves permanently removing parts of the teeth's original structure, including portions that might still be healthy and structurally sound.

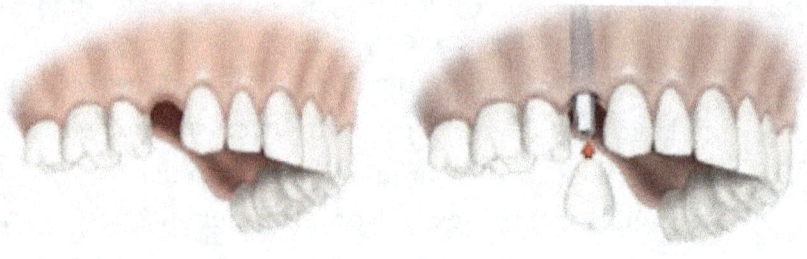

single unit toothless gap   *implant-supported crown*

• *Partial edentulism with the back (posterior) tooth missing*

These conditions imply the absence of several posterior teeth (molars, or molars and premolars) on one or both sides of the dental arch (Kennedy class 1 or Kennedy class 2 Partial Edentulism).

What is *Kennedy class 1 Partial Edentulism*?

> • **Back teeth on both sides of the dental arch are missing. The condition is caused by the early loss of posterior teeth on both sides of the dental arch.**

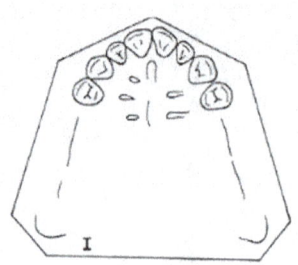

What is *Kennedy class 2 Partial Edentulism*?

• **Posterior teeth on just one side of the dental arch are missing. This condition results from the early loss of molars and premolars on one side of the dental arch.**

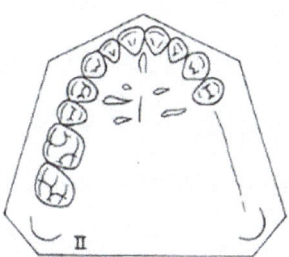

Traditional dental bridges (supported by natural teeth) are challenging to design in these cases because the back support tooth is missing. Removable partial dentures generally require the preparation of 4 to 6 teeth.

Implant-supported restorations (either fixed or removable), although entailing a higher cost, are the best choice in these clinical situations.

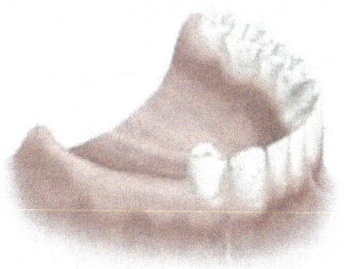

back teeth missing

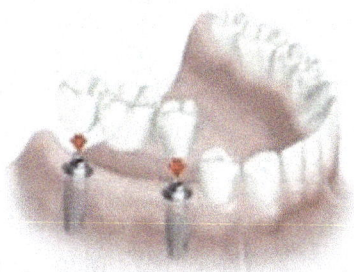

implant-supported bridge

• Complete edentulism

When all teeth are missing, the only traditional solution available is a full removable denture (also known as complete denture). Implant-supported prostheses (either fixed or removable) allow you to chew food better, speak more clearly, and have superior stability.

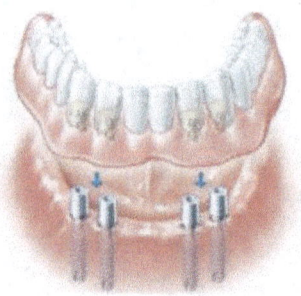 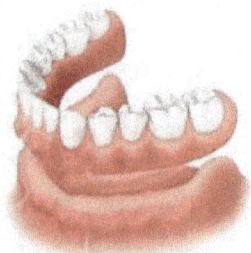

implant-supported denture   *complete denture*

• Other situations when dental implants are highly indicated

> • Patients who cannot tolerate a removable restoration (removable denture).
> • Patients with high aesthetic and functional demands.

General and Local Contraindications

Sometimes, some general or local conditions may prevent the placement of dental implants. Some of these conditions may be addressed before the implant's surgical placement, while others may make the overall placement inadvisable.

Let's review the general and local contraindications for dental implants.

General contraindications

a. Absolute contraindications

Some severe general conditions make anesthesia, surgical procedures, and the overall placement inadvisable.

- Heart diseases affecting the valves, recent infarcts, severe cardiac insufficiency, cardiomyopathy
- Active cancer, certain bone diseases (osteomalacia, Paget's disease, brittle bones syndrome, etc.)
- Certain immunological diseases, immuno-suppressant treatments, clinical AIDS, awaiting an organ transplant
- Certain mental diseases
- Strongly irradiated jaw bones (radiotherapy treatment)
- Treatments of osteoporosis or some cancers by *bisphosphonates*

b. Relative contraindications

Other situations will be evaluated on a case-by-case basis. Most often, dental implants can only be placed (with the greatest caution) after some preliminary treatments.

- Diabetes (particularly insulin-dependent)
- Angina pectoris (angina)
- Significant consumption of tobacco
- Certain mental diseases
- Certain auto-immune diseases
- Drug and alcohol dependency
- Pregnancy

Age

• Children: not before the jaw bones have stopped growing (generally 17-18 years).

• On the other hand, advanced age does not pose problems if the patient's general condition is good.

Local contraindications

Some conditions or physiological changes, usually inside the mouth cavity, may temporarily prevent the placement of dental implants. Most of the time, these conditions can be remedied before the implants are inserted in the jawbone.

• There is insufficient bone to support the implants, or bone structure is inadequate (due to some chronic infections or other conditions). Dental implants must be surrounded by healthy bone tissue to ensure a good prognosis.

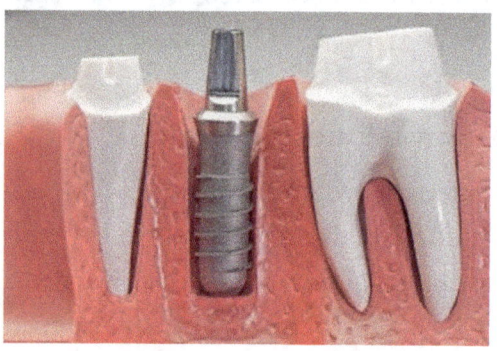

a dental implant must be surrounded by healthy bone tissue (with red)

• Important anatomical structures such as the maxillary sinus or the inferior alveolar nerve (located inside the mandible) have an abnormal position that can interfere with   the dental implants.

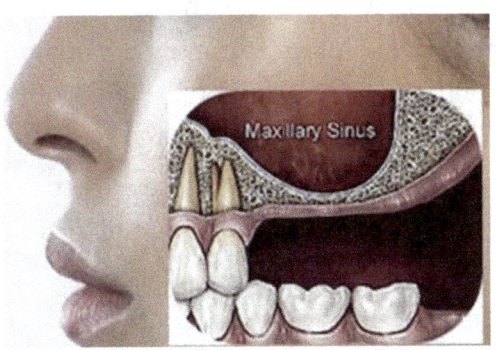

lowering of the maxillary sinus

Adjunctive surgical procedures are crucial in these cases. These procedures aim to increase the amount of bone so that more bone is available to support the implants. We will discuss these procedures later in this book.

• Some local diseases of the oral mucosa or alveolar bone can temporarily prevent the placement of dental implants until the conditions are treated.

• Hypersensitivity or other allergic reactions; fortunately, they rarely occur.

• Poor oral hygiene.

• Bruxism or involuntary grinding of the teeth.

2.4 Dental Implants Vs. Dental Bridges

In the previous chapter, we learned that dental implants often offer the best clinical solution for replacing missing teeth.

This chapter will compare traditional dental bridges supported by natural teeth to dental implant restorations. You will discover the pros and cons of each type of reconstruction and the most important factors to consider when deciding between implants and dental bridges.

You can either get a dental bridge or rely on dental implants to replace lost teeth.

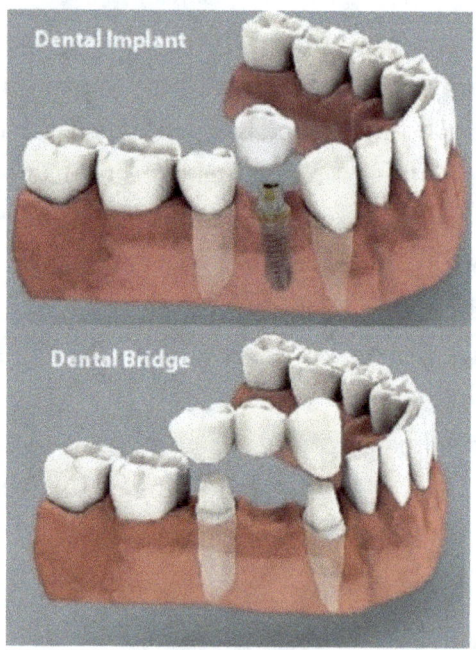

Moreover, if you have a badly damaged tooth, you can either restore it with a dental crown or extract it and place an implant.

In the past, when implants were not available, these decisions were easier to make.

Nowadays, dental implants offer a highly efficient and reliable option; however, you should discuss the advantages and disadvantages of both procedures with your dentist before making your final decision.

a. Replacing lost teeth

Most dentists agree that implants are preferable to fixed bridges in case of missing teeth, assuming the patient has adequate financial ability and time for the entire treatment.

However, there are times when the advantages of a fixed bridge may suggest that a fixed bridge would be preferable to using implants.

First, let's review some general considerations about both procedures:

• *Dental implants*

Dental implants are metal devices surgically inserted into the jawbone to replace one or more missing teeth. Implants can support a dental prosthesis such as a crown, bridge, or removable denture.

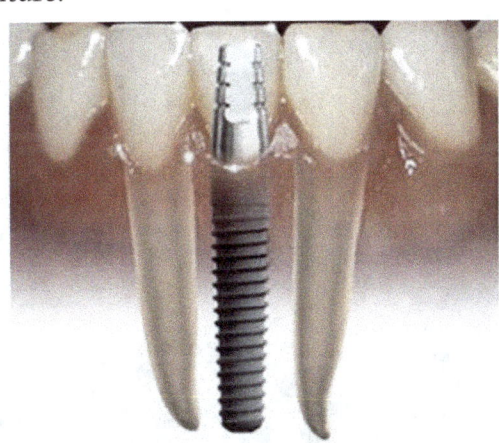

First, a surgical procedure is required to place the dental implant inside the jawbone. Dental implants form an intimate bond with the bone through a biological process called osseointegration.

A variable amount of healing time is required for osseointegration (3 to 6 months), although some approaches aim to shorten this time. We have an entire chapter dedicated to *Same-day Dental Implants*.

After the healing time, an abutment is attached to the implant. The abutment will hold the dental prosthesis (in this case, a dental bridge).

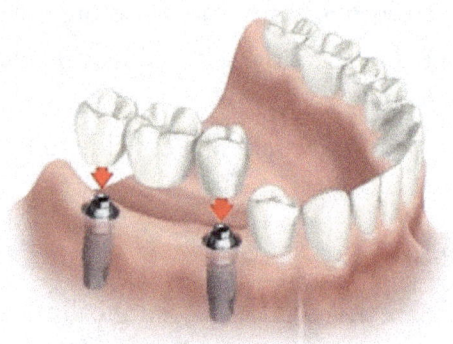

implant-supported dental bridge

• Dental bridge

A dental bridge is a fixed dental prosthesis that replaces one or several missing teeth by permanently joining an artificial tooth to adjacent teeth.

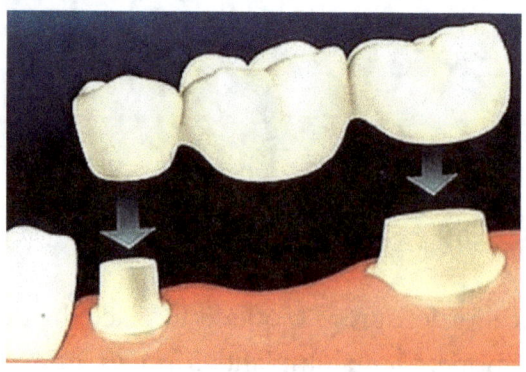

Dental bridges require proper preparation of the adjacent teeth. It is the most significant disadvantage of bridges as it leads to the loss of large amounts of healthy tooth tissue and sometimes even tooth devitalization and endodontic treatment.

Deciding between implants and bridges

It would be best if you always made the decision after consulting with your dentist. They will inform you about the different solutions, advantages, and disadvantages of each, the difference in costs, and any risks and potential complications.

That being said, here are the most important factors to consider:

• *Cost*

> The cost of dental implants is usually higher than a dental bridge; this is especially true if the gap has 2 or 3 missing teeth, in which case you will need more than one implant to restore it.
>
> Moreover, dental implants may need adjunctive procedures (such as sinus lift or bone graft) to increase the amount of bone that supports the implants; these procedures will add to the final cost.

• *Completion time*

> A dental bridge can be completed in two sessions; dental implants generally need more time (3 to 6 months) to fuse with the bone after the surgical procedure.
>
> Nevertheless, in some circumstances, an implant can be placed immediately after a tooth extraction. Still, even in this event, many practitioners will prefer to place temporary restorations for a particular time.

• *Aesthetics*

What about aesthetics? There isn't always a simple answer; typically, dental implants provide the most pleasing results, but a properly constructed ceramic bridge can also be highly aesthetic.

There are times when a cosmetic dentist may prefer a porcelain bridge over an implant because it can give him more control over eliminating the small gaps between teeth that may look unattractive if a dental implant is used.

• *Protecting the adjacent teeth*

Here, dental implants have a significant advantage as they preserve natural tooth tissue by avoiding the need to prepare adjacent teeth. In addition, dental implants offer independent support to crowns and bridges, thus not putting any strain on other teeth.

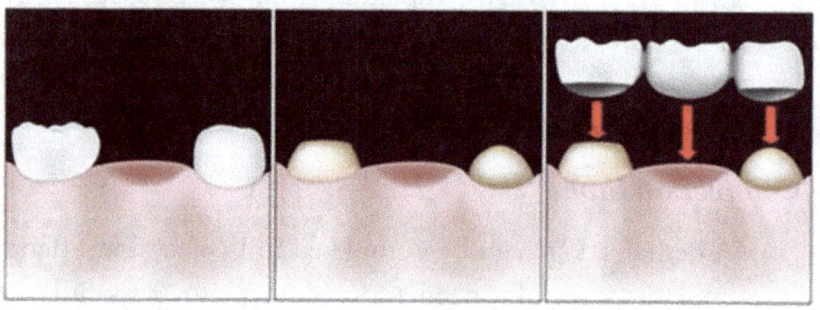

*single tooth gap: if a traditional dental bridge is designed,
the preparation of the adjacent teeth is required*

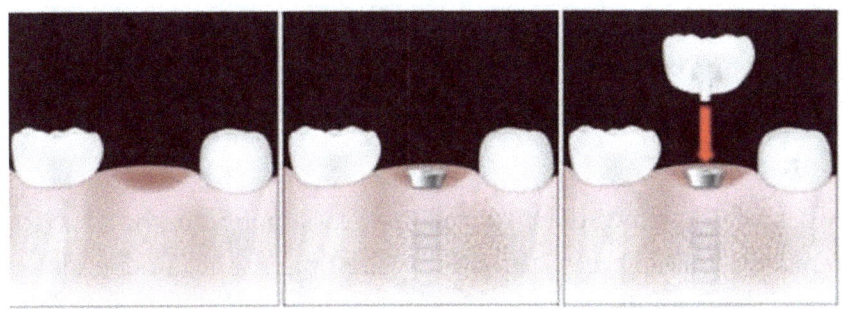

single tooth gap: if an implant-supported crown is manufactured, the adjacent teeth remain untouched

Dental bridges, on the other hand, rely on natural teeth to perform the function of support. After preparation, your natural teeth remain beneath the bridge; hence, the remaining tooth structure continues to be susceptible to decay and gum disease.

• **Maintenance**

Implants are easier to maintain. They can replace teeth individually without affecting other teeth, making regular home care more successful. You can effectively brush and floss around an implant just like your natural tooth.

Dental bridges involve at least three crowns connected together to fill the missing tooth's space. This design creates challenges when brushing and flossing, requiring extra oral hygiene instructions.

• **Durability**

A dental implant, if correctly done, rarely will need replacement. Dental implants are made of solid metal (titanium) and are very resistant to decay and gum problems. The lifespan for the implant-supported bridge is 10 to 15 years.

On the other hand, the average life of a dental bridge is approximately 10 years.

Conclusions

Most of the time, dental implants are superior to bridges for replacing missing teeth. However, the final solution depends on the patient's budget, goals, lifestyle choices, and time restraints.

When might dental bridges be considered the preferred solution?

These situations will be evaluated case-by-case; you should always decide after consulting your dentist.

• If you already have crowns on either side of the missing tooth, then placing a 3-unit bridge may be preferable because it would avoid any surgeries, and the result is that the three teeth would all match.

• If the neighboring teeth have large fillings or extensive structural damage and need crowns in the future.

• If you are a heavy smoker, have untreated periodontal disease, or have a large bony defect.

• If you do not have the budget to have an implant placed or cannot return to the clinic for the definitive implant restoration.

b. Restoring a damaged tooth

When a large part of a tooth's original crown structure has been lost, you can either restore the tooth with a dental crown (left image) or extract the tooth and place an implant. The implant will then support the dental crown (right image).

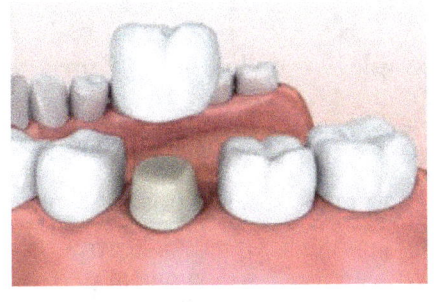 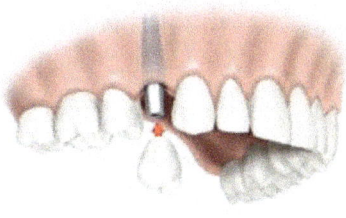

The decision should be based on:
- the amount of tooth structure remaining
- the type of occlusion (or bite)
- financial considerations
- patient desire to keep the natural tooth
- patient acceptance of other needed procedures to retain the tooth, such as a root canal and sometimes the placement of a *post and core*.

What is a *Post and Core*?

• A post and core is a prosthetic device utilized when inadequate tooth structure remains to support a traditional restoration or an artificial crown.

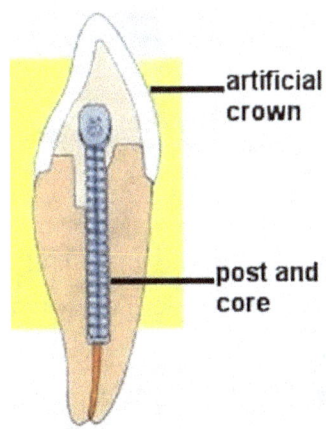

artificial crown

post and core

The post is a small rod, usually metal, inserted into the tooth's root space and protruding a couple of millimeters from the root.

The post is then used to hold the core in place.

Because the post is inserted into the root canal, a post and core can only be made for a tooth that has had root canal treatment.

The core replaces the missing tooth structure in preparation for a new dental crown.

The core is generally made of metal alloys and holds the dental crown in place.

It is a good idea to save the tooth whenever the procedure is possible.

However, when the tooth crown is severely damaged, mainly when the tooth is fractured below the gumline, removing the tooth and placing a dental implant is the only solution.

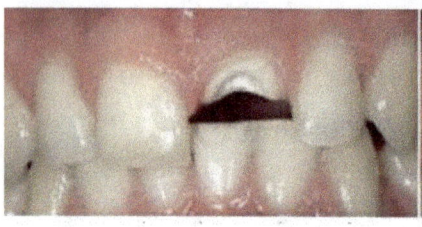 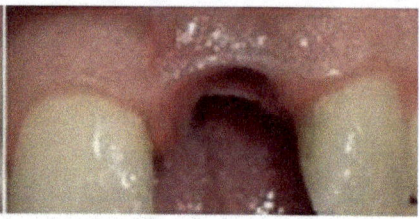

a case when the tooth can be restored with a post and a dental crown

tooth with advanced coronal destructions; extraction and placement of dental implant indicated

In the first situation, a post and core will be inserted into the tooth's root space, and then a dental crown will be constructed to replace the missing tooth.

The post and core will hold the dental crown in place.

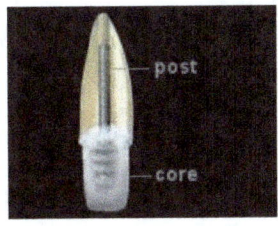 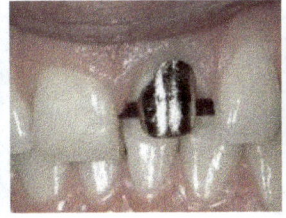 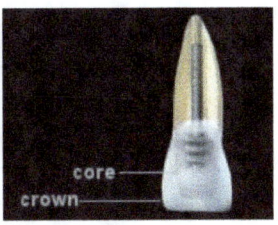

In the second case, after the tooth's removal, the implant crown can either be manufactured with the traditional procedure (which can take up to one year) or using a *same-day implant* if the clinical situation is suitable.

More details about this procedure are in the "*Same-day dental implants*" chapter.

2.5 Dental Implants Cost

The cost of dental implants depends on many factors, including the type of implantation, the type of prosthetic reconstruction, the dentist performing the procedure, the location where the implant placement surgery and the prosthetic phase are carried out, the dental implant material used, and the amount of dental insurance.

You can only find out the exact cost of an implant-supported restoration after a complete medical examination.

That being said, here are some general price considerations about dental implants. Always discuss with your dentist the various types of implant-supported reconstructions available and their prices.

Most of the time, a dental implant reconstruction requires multiple procedures, and the final cost results by adding the costs of these procedures together.

- a. Dental implant procedure
- b. Prosthetic device placement
- c. Adjunctive surgical procedures - required in some situations to increase the amount of bone

We have detailed information about these procedures and devices, so check the appropriate chapters for more details.

a. Dental implant

Dental implants are surgically inserted into the alveolar bone. The total number of implants required for a particular situation depends on the type of prosthetic restoration and the number of missing teeth.

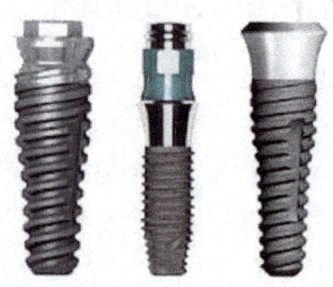

dental implants of various shapes and sizes

Single implants may range in cost from $400 to $4,000, depending on multiple factors:

- the type of implantation
- the dentist performing the procedure
- the location where the operation is performed; price can vary a lot in different parts of the world
- the dental implant material used
- the amount of dental insurance

b. Prosthetic device

There is a large diversity of prosthetic devices that can be constructed on dental implants. Usually, when many teeth are missing, the implant reconstruction will be more expensive than in the case of small toothless gaps.

• Dental crown

An implant-supported crown is a small reconstruction generally used when a single tooth is missing.

Typically, implant-supported crowns are made of porcelain fused to metal alloys (gold, titanium, etc.), zirconia, or all ceramics.

We have an entire section about what implant-supported restorations are made of.

The price depends on the type of crown; zirconia or gold-based crowns are more expensive.

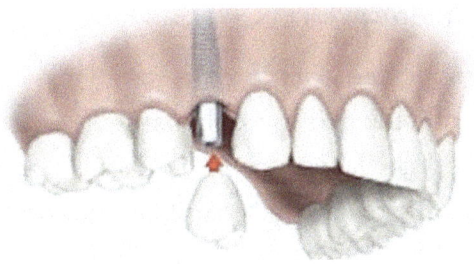

implant-supported crown

• Fixed dental bridge

A fixed dental bridge supported by implants is generally indicated when several teeth (or all teeth) are missing.

More implants are needed to support a bridgework restoration than an implant-supported removable denture.

Similar to dental crowns, the price of a bridgework reconstruction usually depends on the material used but may also vary based on other factors.

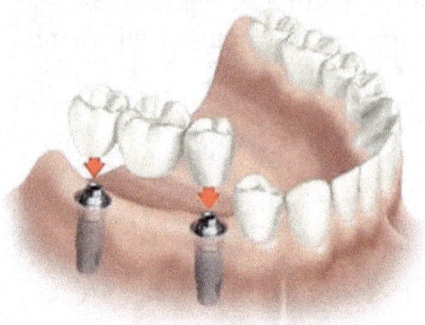

implant-supported bridge

Most often, the cost of a fixed restoration (crown, bridge) supported by dental implants is more expensive than the same type of restoration supported by natural teeth (traditional restoration).

• *Removable denture*

An implant-supported denture is a type of overdenture supported by and attached to implants.

An implant-supported denture is used when a person doesn't have any teeth in the jaw. An implant-supported denture has special attachments that snap onto attachments on the implants.

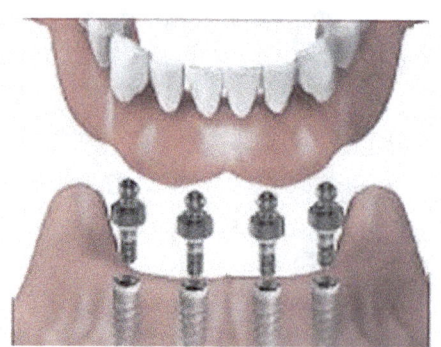

implant-supported denture

You should remove your denture daily to clean the denture and gum area. However, implant-supported dentures allow one to chew food better, speak more clearly, and have superior stability compared to traditional dentures.

Because of the many types of implant-supported dentures available, your healthcare provider can only estimate the price after the medical examination.

c. Adjunctive surgical procedures

In some situations, the size or structure of the bone is not adequate to support dental implants. Adjunctive surgical procedures aim to increase the amount of bone so more bone is available to support the implants.

Some procedures seek to recreate the soft tissues (gingival tissue) or to reposition anatomical structures that might interfere with the dental implants.

The cost will be significantly higher if laborious operations are required (complex bone reconstruction, sinus lift). However, a dental implant must be surrounded by healthy bone tissue to ensure a long-term success rate.

Consequently, if there is a lack of bone, these procedures are essential before the implant placement.

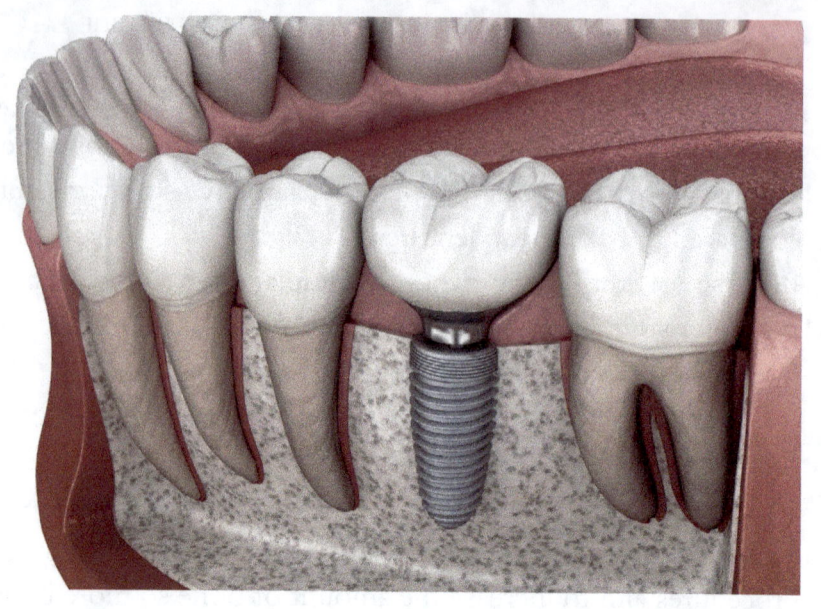

3. Dental Implant Structure

♦♦♦

A dental implant restoration consists of 3 main parts:

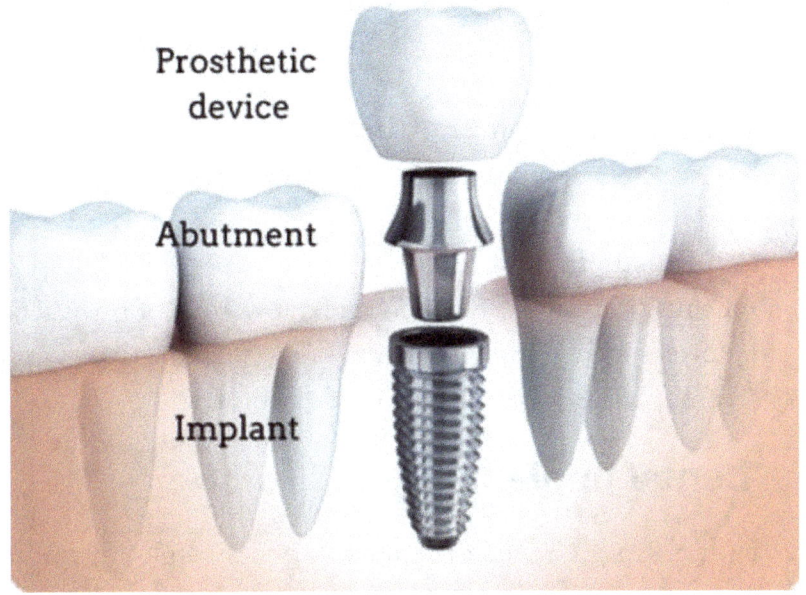

Prosthetic
device

Abutment

Implant

1. Dental implant

A surgical component that interfaces with the bone of the jaw or skull to support a dental prosthesis, such as a crown, bridge, or removable denture.

A surgical procedure is required to place the dental implant inside the jawbone. One or more implants may be necessary for a specific case.

For example, a single implant will be positioned when a tooth is missing. If all teeth from a dental arch are missing, 4 to 8 implants may be required to support the restoration.

2. Abutment

Implant abutments are artificial devices that are connected to the dental implants after the healing process is over.

The abutments are used to attach a crown, bridge, or removable denture to the implant fixtures.

3. Prosthetic device

Dental implants can support a large variety of prosthetic devices: dental crowns, dental bridges, and various types of implant-supported removable dentures.

3.1 Dental Implant

Dental implants are metal or zirconia devices surgically inserted into the jawbone.

Structure

Dental implants come in a variety of shapes and sizes, so there is one to suit every clinical situation. An implant is actually an "artificial tooth root"; the implant surface is ribbed for better integration into bone tissue.

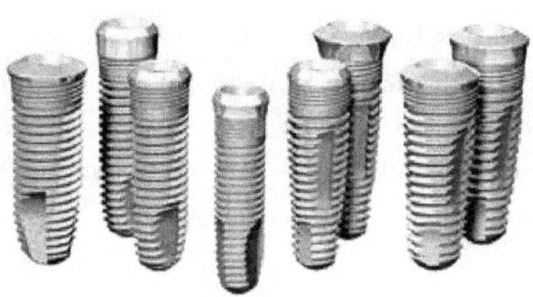

dental implants

Implants are also threaded; when screwed into the bone, they collect bone tissue so that the implant is as stable as possible when it integrates into the bone.

Some implants are moulded as one piece with the crown; in this case, the type of the crown is pre-determined. More often, an abutment is attached to the implant after the healing period; this allows for more fine-tuning.

Manufacturing material

In most cases, dental implants are made of titanium. Titanium is the most favored material by most dental clinicians and implant manufacturing companies due to its high biocompatibility, non-allergic and tissue-friendly nature, and its remarkable ability to make a connection of its surface with the alveolar bone for the process of osseointegration.

In addition, zirconia dental implants have recently emerged. Even though they are relatively new, there has been a considerable increase in the use of these dental implants. More about zirconia dental implants in the following subchapter.

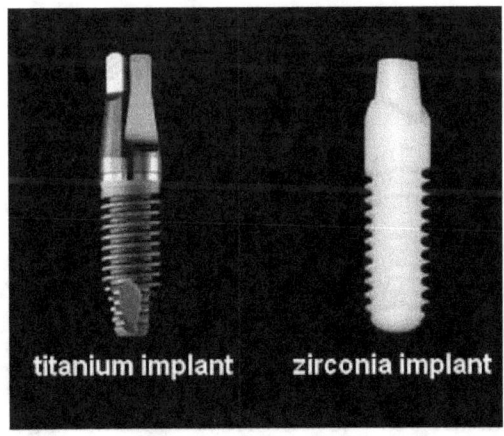

titanium implant   zirconia implant

Dental implant tool kit

The implantation procedure requires specialized tools. Generally, the manufacturing companies supply the implants along with a specific tool kit.

The dental implant tool kit also contains instruments needed for the surgical procedure and the prosthetic phase. The tool kit is supplied together with dental implants and abutments of various shapes and sizes.

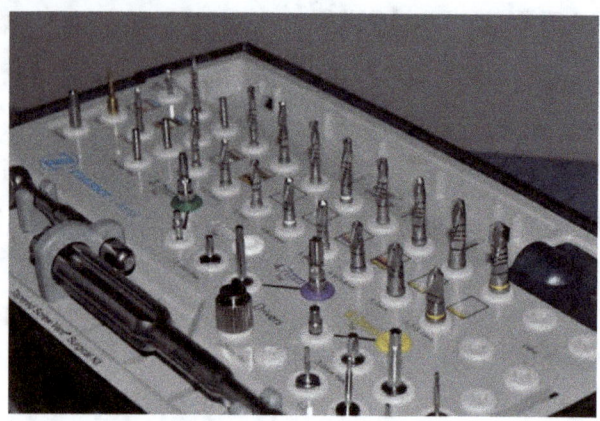

Here is what a kit usually consists of:
- titanium surgical drills of various sizes, color-coded
- implant insertion tools
- insertion tools for artificial abutments and healing abutments
- healing abutments and cover screws; these devices are attached to the implants immediately after the surgical placement
- different screw keys
- *physiodispenser*: a device used for bone cooling during surgery; the bone must always be protected from high temperatures to prevent irreversible damage

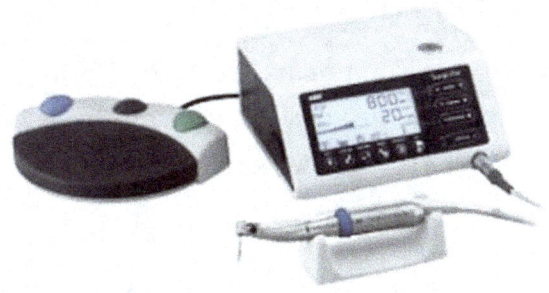

- other supporting elements, may include guide pins, special trays, stents, etc.

3.2 Abutment

Implant abutments are artificial devices connected to the dental implants after the healing process. The abutments are used to attach a crown, bridge, or removable denture to the implant fixtures.

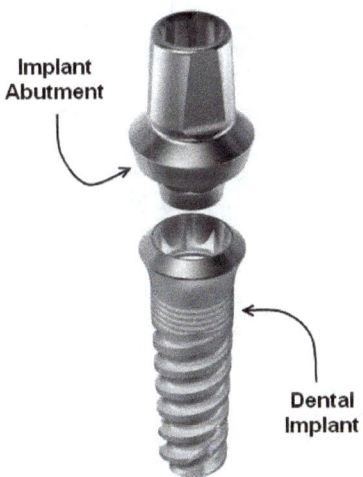

There are two classes of abutments: prefabricated and custom-made.

a. Prefabricated abutments

Prefabricated or stock abutments are manufactured in a range of sizes and shapes and are usually delivered by manufacturing companies along with the implants.

Material

Prefabricated abutments can be made from a variety of materials, such as titanium, surgical stainless steel, gold, and, more recently, zirconia.

• Titanium abutments

Titanium abutments are widely used due to the excellent properties of titanium alloys. They have outstanding strength and biocompatibility and can be used for any type of prosthetic restoration.

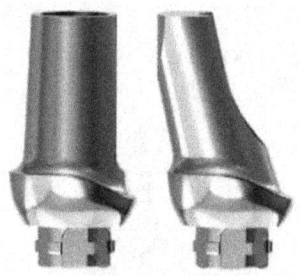

titanium abutments

Most clinicians feel more comfortable using a metal prosthetic abutment in the posterior molar areas due to the increased masticatory forces.

• Zirconia abutments

Zirconia abutments are more modern abutments and are used better to complement the aesthetics of dental implant restorations.

When all ceramics or zirconia restorations are planned, zirconia implant abutments provide a highly desirable option. When a zirconia abutment is used, the problem of matching the shade of adjacent teeth while hiding the dark color of the metal abutment is avoided.

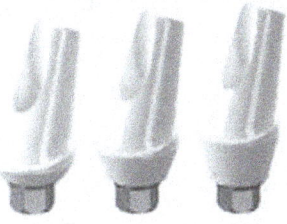

zirconia abutments

Moreover, in 2011, a one-piece zirconia implant (fixture and abutment) was introduced into the market.

• Other materials

Besides titanium and zirconia, artificial abutments can be made of gold alloy, stainless steel, or other metal alloys. Although indications are narrower, there are situations in which these may be successfully utilized.

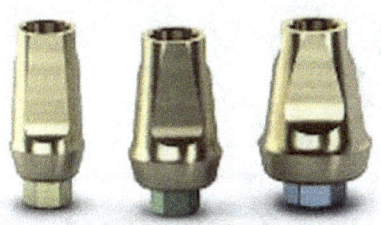

gold abutments

How is an implant abutment selected?

When the practitioner selects the abutments, several factors are involved:

> • The position of the implant: larger artificial abutments are positioned in the back of the mouth due to the increased chewing forces
>
> • The type of prosthesis that is executed: crown, fixed bridge, or removable denture; special retainer-type abutments are used to secure implant-supported dentures
>
> • How the restoration is attached to the abutments: with dental cement, with lag screws, or with special retainers

Let's examine these factors in more detail:

I. The prosthesis is secured to the abutments with dental cement

In this case, the surface of the artificial abutment is smooth. The restoration is connected to the abutments with dental cement, just like crowns and bridges are fixed on natural teeth.

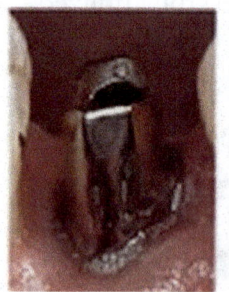 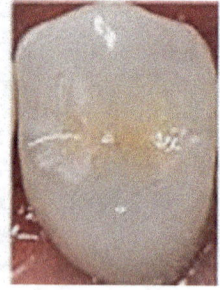

abutment and implant-supported crown secured with dental cement

The main advantage is they offer a higher aesthetic performance.

II. The prosthesis is fixed with a lag screw

These restorations require artificial abutments with a threaded hole in the middle.

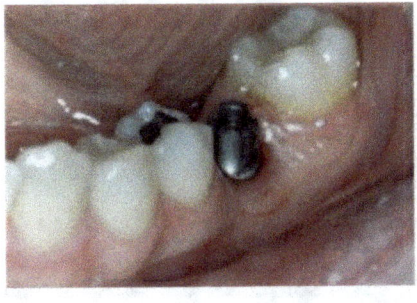 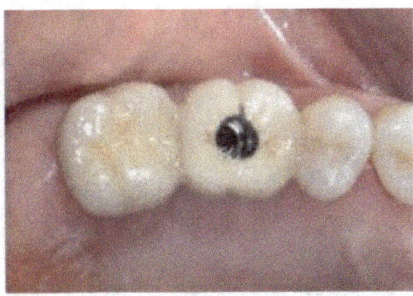

artificial abutment with a threaded hole   *the crown is secured with a lag-screw*

The restoration is secured with screws that traverse the dental crowns and attach to the threaded holes. After the screws are positioned, the holes that penetrate the crowns are sealed with a composite material.

The advantage is they are easier to maintain and change when the prosthetic fractures.

III. Removable dentures secured with special retainers

Special retainer-type abutments are used to retain dentures using a *male-adapter* attached to the implant and a *female-adapter* in the denture.

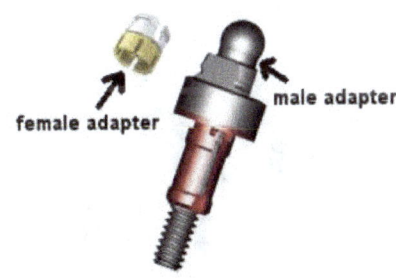 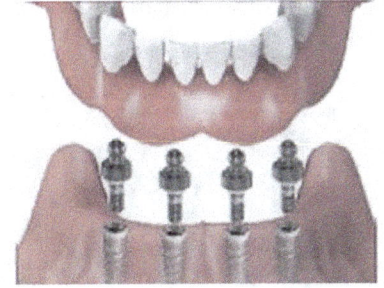

male-adapter and female-adapter   *implant-supported denture*

Compared to conventional dentures, these abutments allow movement of the denture but enough retention to improve the quality of life for denture wearers.

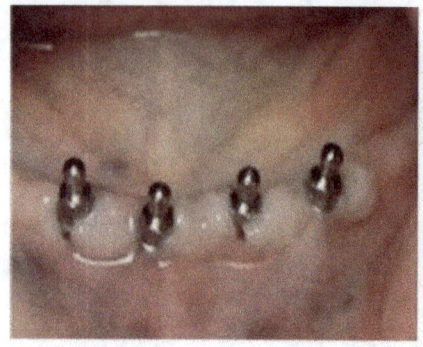 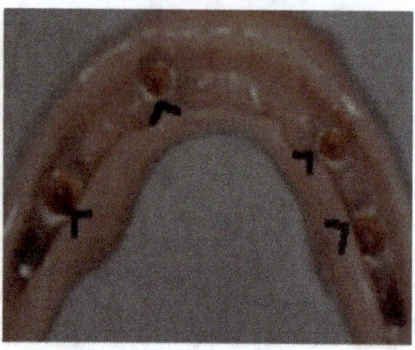

the male-adapters
are attached to the implants

the female-adapters
are housed in the denture

Regardless of the type of adapter, the female portion of the adapter housed in the denture will require periodic replacement.

Angulation

An abutment is not necessarily parallel to the long axis of the implant. Angulated abutments are utilized when the implant is at a different inclination in relation to the proposed prosthesis.
In this case, the primary purpose is to make all artificial abutments parallel.

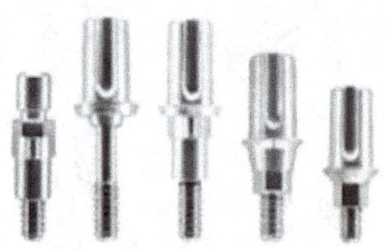 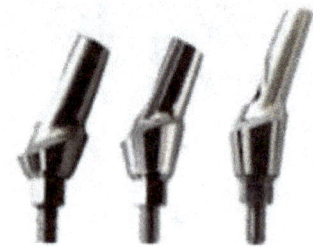

straight abutments

angulated abutments

b. Custom-made abutments

Custom-made abutments are fabricated at the dental laboratory after a dental impression of the top of the implant is made with the adjacent teeth and gingiva. The size, shape, and material depend on the clinical application.

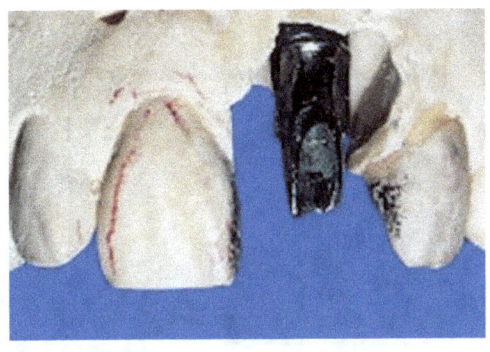

custom-made abutment on a dental cast

What is a *Dental Impression*?

• A *traditional dental impression* is an imprint of teeth and soft tissues formed with specific impression materials used in different dentistry areas. The dental impression forms an imprint (i.e., a 'negative' mould) of teeth and soft tissues, which can then be used to create a cast of the dentition.

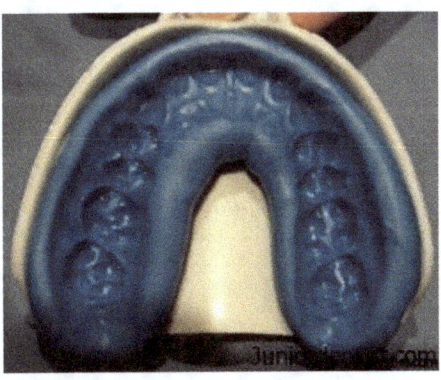

• **A digital dental impression is a cutting-edge technology that enables dentists to build a computer-generated, virtual replica of the soft and hard tissues in the mouth. Digital impressions are created with optical scanning devices such as lasers.**

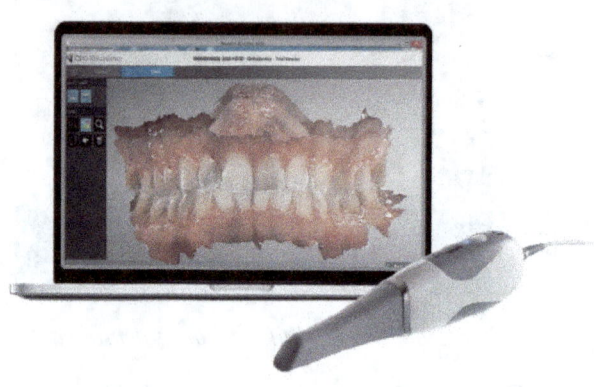

Commonly, any abutment can be manufactured at the dental lab: with a smooth surface, threaded holes, and anchoring systems for removable dentures.

Another variation is when the crown and abutment are one piece, and the lag screw traverses both to secure the one-piece structure to the internal thread on the implant.

Regardless of the type of abutment, after the abutment is attached to the implant, an impression is made, and the designed restoration is constructed at the dental laboratory (for more details, see the *prosthetic phase*).

3.2.1 Zirconia Implants

As we have seen, a dental implant restoration consists of 3 main parts: dental implant, abutment, and prosthetic device. In this chapter, we'll discuss the first two parts: the dental implant and the abutment.

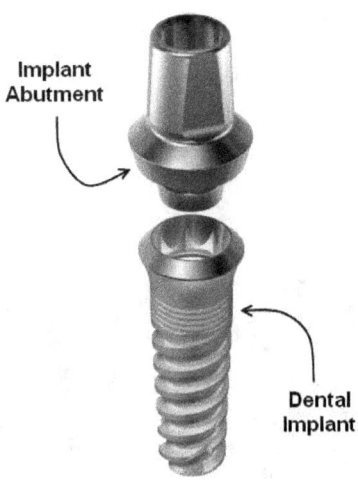

Initially, both these parts were made of titanium. Titanium was (and still is) the most favored material by most dental clinicians and implant manufacturing companies due to its high biocompatibility.

a. Titanium implant fixture with zirconia abutment

The improvements in new ceramic materials made it possible to have the abutment part made of a special kind of white ceramic called zirconia.

Although pure zirconium is technically a metal (based on its location on the periodic table), the crystalline form used for dental implants and dental restorations (known as zirconia) is more similar to ceramic, so it doesn't act like a metal in the mouth.

Zirconia is commonly known to be more tissue-friendly than titanium, providing better aesthetics. In this variation, the implant fixture is still made of titanium.

b. All zirconia implants

The next step was to develop a complete zirconia implant. In 2011, a one-piece zirconia implant (fixture and abutment) was introduced into the market. Even though relatively new, there has been a considerable increase in the use of these types of implants.

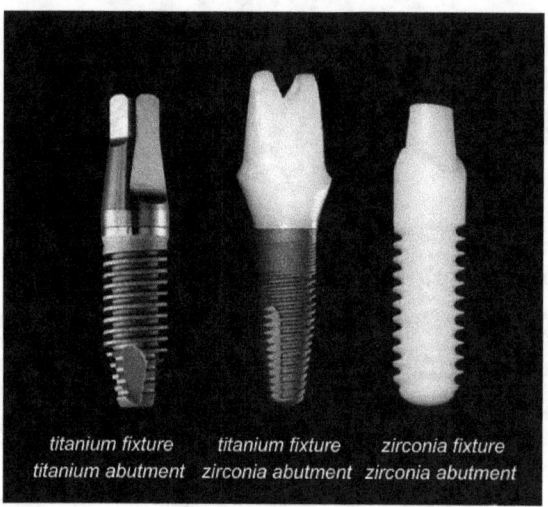

titanium fixture   titanium fixture   zirconia fixture
titanium abutment zirconia abutment zirconia abutment

Zirconia implants benefits

• One of the main advantages of a one-piece zirconia implant is that it has no prosthetic connections, where bacteria can grow, and therefore can lead to better gum health.

• Because zirconia is white, it is more aesthetically pleasing and natural-looking. In this case, the entire implant restoration will be metal-free, so the problem of matching the shade of adjacent teeth while hiding the dark color of the metal abutment is avoided.

• Gums are healthier around ceramic materials and better preserved. Because no metal is involved, the color of the gums will remain natural-pink.

• Another quality of zirconia is its resistance to corrosion, which, theoretically, does not apply to titanium. Being a metal, titanium can be subjected to corrosion, although this is highly unlikely.

• Zirconia implants are hypoallergenic, giving patients with titanium allergies (which are extremely rare) an alternative for dental implants.

Drawbacks and concerns

The main problem with zirconia implants is the need for studies examining the chemical and structural composition and the level of osseointegration achieved with zirconia implants.

The studies conducted so far do not allow for the recommendation of the use of zirconia implants in daily practice. However, zirconia dental implants have the potential to become a viable alternative to titanium implants, but they are not yet in routine clinical use.

Conclusion

There is no question that titanium implants have the best long-term data to support their use. The data on zirconia implants is much more limited. However, zirconia implants have certain advantages, such as superior aesthetics and better gum health around them, but it is not clear how well they integrate with the bone.

3.3 Implant-Supported Prostheses

Dental implants can support a large variety of prosthetic devices. When planning for a type of implant-supported restoration, several factors are involved:

- The number and position of missing teeth
- The overall clinical conditions
- Aesthetic and functional demands
- Geographical location: different types of prostheses can be designed in various parts of the world
- Whether a patient can afford the designed solution
- The expertise and preferences of each practitioner

a. Dental crown

An implant-supported crown is typically indicated when a single tooth is missing. However, it is possible to design adjacent single-unit crowns when several teeth are missing.

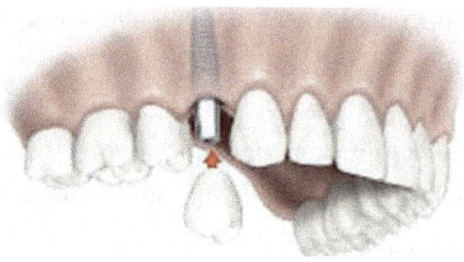

Dental crowns can be made of porcelain fused to metal alloys (gold, titanium, base metals), zirconia, or all ceramics. Execution time is relatively short, and the success rate is excellent.

b. Dental bridge

Many patients prefer fixed implant-supported bridges because they do not have to be removed for cleaning. Bridges are permanently secured on the implants either with dental cement or with lag screws. Large dental bridges supported by many implants can be quite expensive.

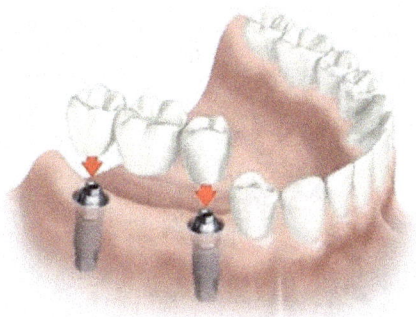

It is not advisable to design dental bridges supported by both natural teeth and dental implants, as this could lead to the loosening of the implants because of natural teeth' physiological mobility and failure.

What does *natural teeth' physiological mobility* mean?

> • **Natural teeth are intended to have a little mobility. This is because the tooth is not fused to the bones of the jaws but is connected to the sockets by the flexible periodontal ligament.**
>
> **This ligament allows the tooth to move just slightly, but people should not actually be able to see or feel this movement.**

Let's detail the above idea:
Contrary to natural teeth, dental implants fuse to the bone and, as a result, have no mobility at all. Consequently, the natural

mobility of the tooth causes the chewing forces to act as a lever on the rigid implant fixture.

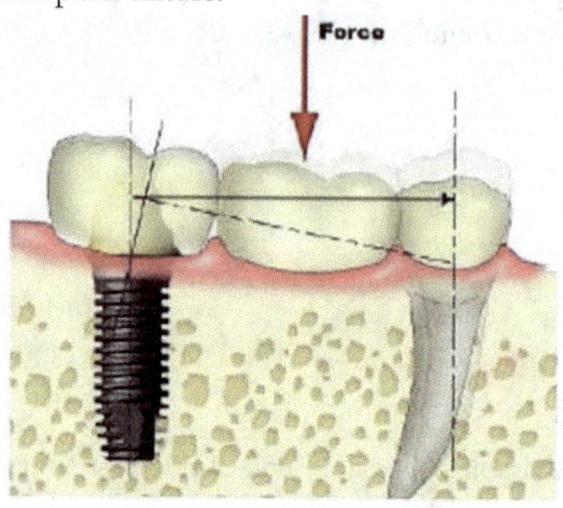

this graphic shows an implant
in a bridge connection with a natural tooth

Moreover, designing enough implant units to adequately support the bridge is equally important. For example, if all teeth are missing and a fixed dental bridge is designed, at least six implants are required to support the bridgework.

Even in the case of *All-on-4 dental implants*, many practitioners prefer to place a few extra implants as an extra precaution.

What is an *All-on-4 system*?

> • The term All-on-4 refers to 'all' teeth being supported 'on four' dental implants, a prosthodontics procedure for total rehabilitation of a toothless dental arch.

c. Dentures

An implant-supported denture is a type of overdenture supported by and attached to implants. An implant-supported denture should be removed daily to clean the denture and gum area.

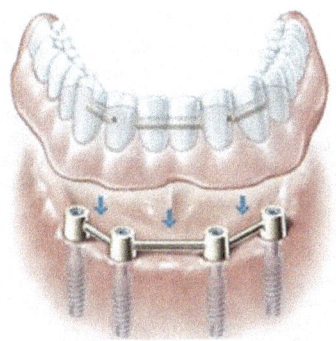

Compared to a traditional denture (complete denture), which rests exclusively on the gums, implant-supported dentures allow chewing the food better and speaking more clearly. Moreover, they have superior stability.

Removable dentures are generally designed when all teeth from a dental arch are missing. When a removable denture is worn, **retainers** to hold the denture in place are attached to the implants and the denture.

Special retainers

Most often, the retainers are made of two components:

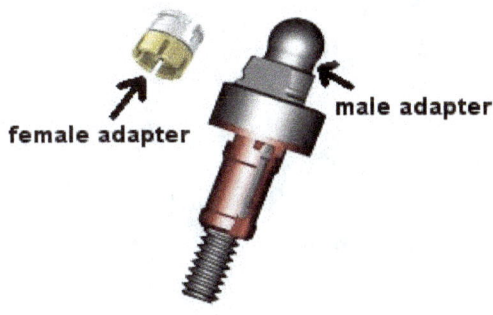

- A **male-adapter** - attached to the implant
- A **female adapter** - housed in the denture. This part will require periodic replacement.

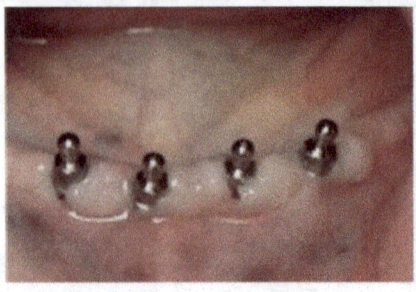 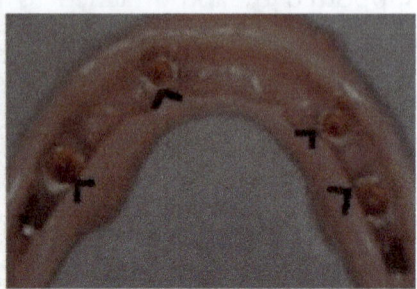

the male-adapters
are attached to the implants

the female-adapters
are housed in the denture

Various adapters are designed to hold overdentures in place, for example, the ball-and-socket style retainer (image above) or the button-style adapter.

Another variation is when a cast bar of metal is secured to the implants. The complete denture then attaches to the bar with attachments, allowing no movement of the denture (image below).

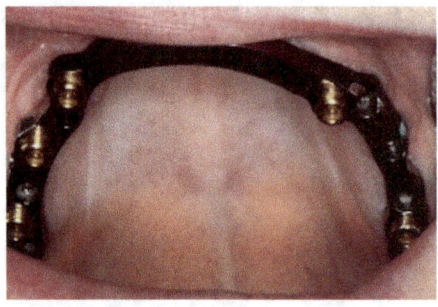

d. Orthodontic anchors

Dental implants can be used as orthodontic anchors to align teeth. Orthodontic implants differ from those used for prosthetics, as there is no osseointegration. Mini-implants provide absolute anchorage, and they have revolutionized the field of orthodontics.

3.3.1 What Are Implant-Supported Restorations Made Of?

Three main types of prostheses can be constructed on dental implants:

- dental crowns
- dental bridges
- dentures

In this chapter, we will discuss an implant restoration structure, the manufacturing materials used, and the advantages and drawbacks of each type.

a. Dental Crowns and Dental Bridges

In the vast majority of cases, porcelain crowns and bridges are preferred when it comes to fixed implant restorations.

Porcelain is superior to any other aesthetic material used in dentistry because of the great aesthetic features that make porcelain restorations look almost like natural teeth.

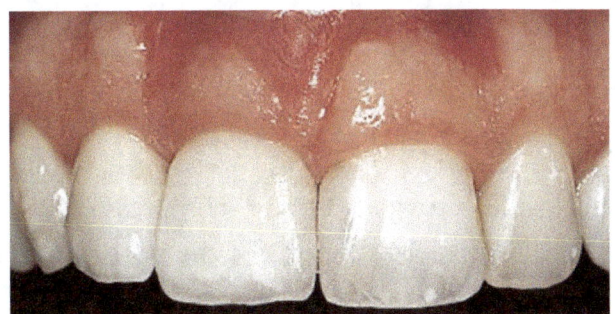

*porcelain crowns on the two central incisors;
notice the outstanding aesthetics*

Several kinds of ceramic restorations may be utilized, and we have detailed information on each.

- Porcelain Fused To Metal Restorations (where the metal frame can be made of base metal alloys, gold, or titanium)
- Porcelain Fused to Zirconia Restorations
- All Ceramics Restorations

I. Porcelain Fused To Metal Restorations

Porcelain fused to metal rehabilitations are widely used in dentistry. They have a metal shell on which porcelain is fused in a high-heat oven.

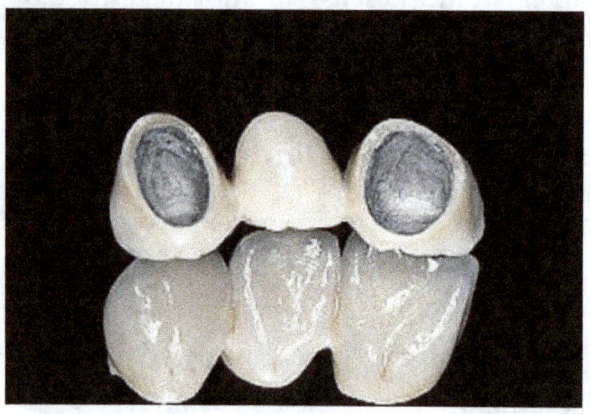

porcelain fused to metal bridge

Structure

*** *Metal frame*

The metal frame provides strong compression and tensile strength as well as proper support for the porcelain that will be fused on it.

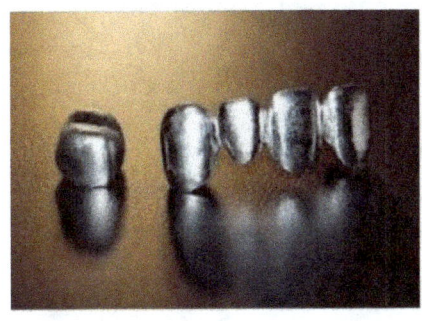 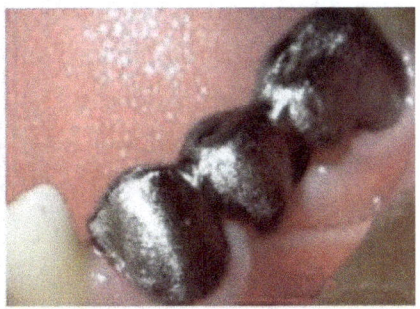

porcelain crown and bridge metal frame   *metal frame inside the mouth cavity*

The metal alloys used in combination with dental ceramics are specific. Their composition allows a powerful chemical bond with the porcelain layer fused on top, which significantly increases the strength of the connection between metal and porcelain.

The quality and price of porcelain fused to metal restorations largely depend on the metal alloy used to manufacture the frame.

• Base metal alloys

These types of alloys have only base metals in their composition. The most common base metals used in dentistry are chromium, nickel, aluminum, iron, or tin.

Although they don't have the same attributes as noble metal alloys (gold, silver, palladium), porcelain fused to base metal alloy reconstructions are solid and durable, and the price is reasonable.

• Titanium alloys

Titanium is a unique base metal alloy with superior qualities.

Titanium alloys are widely used in dentistry, mainly for dental implants, implant abutments, and various types of prosthetic devices.

Titanium alloys are non-allergic, tissue-friendly, strong, and durable. Although titanium-based restorations are more expensive than base-metal ones, they are generally cheaper than gold-based ones.

• Gold alloys

Although referred to as gold alloys, these metal alloys are actually composed of different elements, including gold, platinum, palladium, silver, copper, and tin.

The first four elements listed are noble metals, while the last two are base or non-noble metals. The gold alloy is better quality when it is high in noble content.

Gold alloy develops powerful chemical bonds with the ceramic layer like the other alloys.

- ☐ Dental gold is an alloy that is used only in dentistry.
- ☐ Gold alloys used for ceramic restorations have a specific composition.
- ☐ Gold alloys used for other types of prosthetic devices have a different composition.

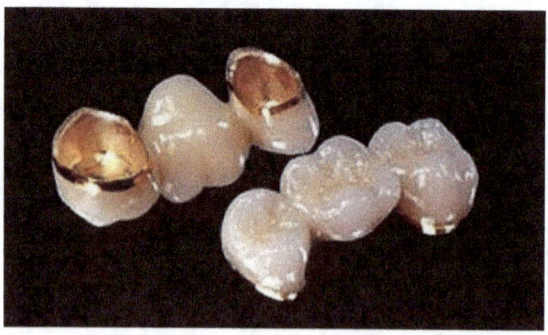

porcelain fused to gold dental bridge

Gold alloys have superior strength and resistance: a gold alloy frame can be manufactured at a shallow thickness and still preserve its high strength and resistance. Moreover, gold alloys are light, have high biocompatibility, and never corrode.

Although these restorations are usually the most expensive, they are superior to the first two types.

*** Porcelain layer

Porcelain can cover the metal core on all sides, leaving no parts of the metal visible.

Another variation is that crowns are made with a *partial veneer* that covers only the visible aspects of the crown, while the remaining surfaces of the crown are bare metal.

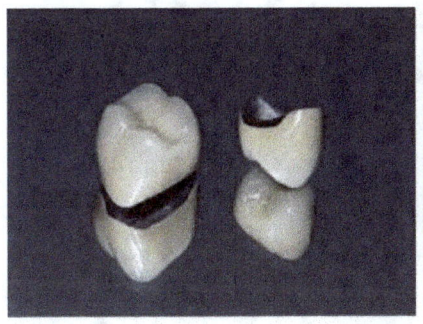 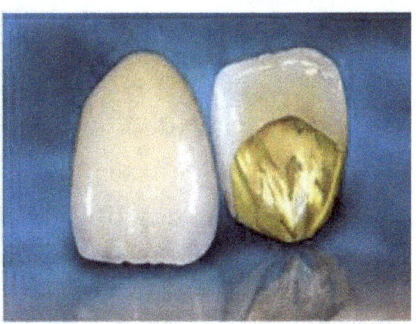

porcelain covers all sides of the metal frame   *crown with a partial veneer*

The first of the two variations has superior aesthetics.

When it comes to dental ceramics, a vast range of colors, with the possibility of combining them, are available. Consequently, porcelain will give the crown a tooth-like appearance and can be color-matched to the adjacent teeth or gingivae.

Moreover, porcelain is a material that has a translucency similar to enamel. This quality significantly enhances its visual appeal.

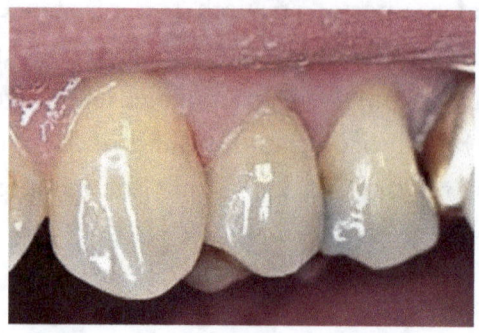

porcelain crown (on the center tooth)
color matched to the adjacent teeth

Does *dental ceramics* mean the same as *dental porcelain*?

• Yes. Both terms describe the same thing.

II. Porcelain Fused To Zirconia Restorations

Zirconia is the hardest-known ceramic in the industry and the strongest material used in dentistry.

The zirconia used in dentistry is *zirconium oxide*, which has been stabilized by adding yttrium oxide.

Zirconia is a firm white ceramic delivered in solid blocks of various shapes and sizes. Processing requires sophisticated computer systems known as CAD/CAM systems. We will discuss CAD/CAM systems in the Laboratory Stages subchapter.

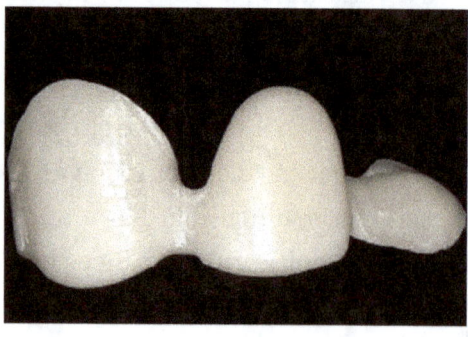

zirconia framework

Zirconia may be used to construct any fixed prosthetic restoration. However, when dental crowns or bridges are entirely manufactured of zirconia ceramic, they will have a white color.

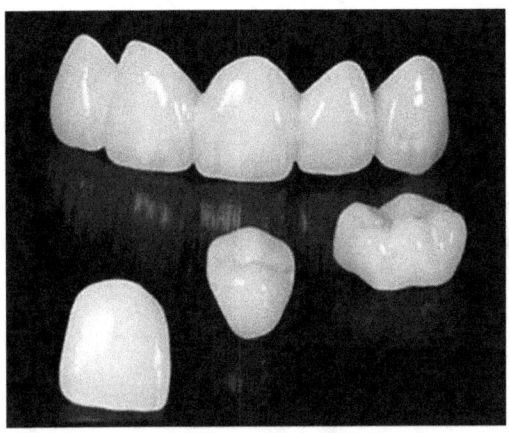

full zirconia crowns and bridges

For this reason, zirconia is most often utilized to manufacture the supporting frame for ceramic restorations. The frame will then be layered with porcelain to give the reconstructions a highly aesthetic appearance.

Features and Benefits

Zirconia is a recently emerged material that has revolutionized dentistry. Because of its exceptional qualities, it can be utilized for various purposes.

• Zirconia is highly durable and tough. It is basically the most robust material used in dentistry to this point.

• Because it is a white ceramic with outstanding translucency features, zirconia-based restorations are highly aesthetic because they do not contain any metal in their structure.

• The zirconia core structure can be layered with aesthetic porcelain to create the final color and shape of the tooth.

• Similar to gold, it has a high biocompatibility, no allergic effects, and, because it is not a metal, it never corrodes.

• Because computer systems execute them, zirconia-based prostheses are highly precise.

• Unfortunately, it is still expensive. Both the material and the necessary processing equipment lead to a high final cost.

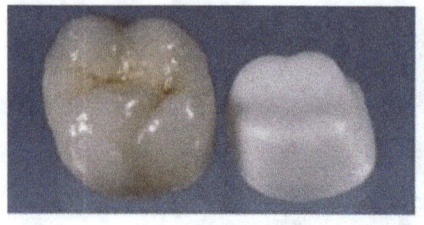 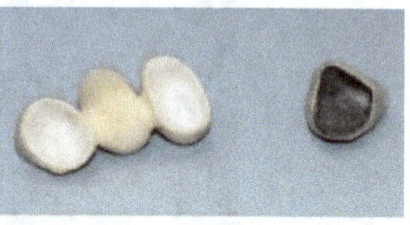

porcelain crown with zirconia substructure   *zirconia and metal frame restorations*

III. All Ceramic Restorations

All ceramic or full porcelain restorations are constructed entirely from porcelain without a metal or zirconia frame. They are particularly indicated when the designed restoration is located in the front area of your mouth, where aesthetic demands are very high.

With no supporting frame, they are less resistant, and therefore, all ceramics are not used in the back area because of the increased chewing forces.

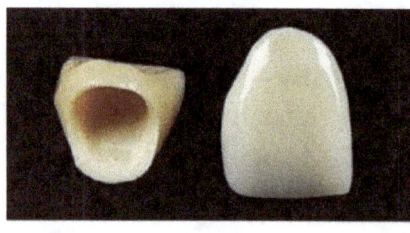 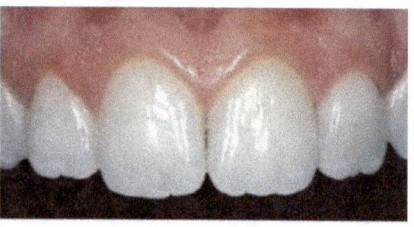

all ceramic crown

all ceramic crowns on both central incisors

• All ceramic restorations are highly aesthetic because they are made entirely of porcelain.

• They do not have the strength of zirconia or metal-based restorations. As a result, case selection must be rigorously conducted.

• Generally, designing full ceramic bridges that exceed 2 or 3 units is not advisable. Because there is no supporting frame, the bridge might break or be irreversibly damaged.

All ceramic crowns are manufactured with computerized systems, and particular types of ceramics are required. Consequently, they are more expensive than porcelain fused to metal reconstructions.

b. Dentures

An implant-supported denture (also known as removable denture or, in some cases, overdenture) is a prosthetic device sustained by dental implants that replaces all teeth from a dental arch.

An implant-supported denture should be removed daily to clean the denture and gum area.

Implant dentures consist of 3 parts:

   • the base
   • the artificial teeth
   • the special retainers

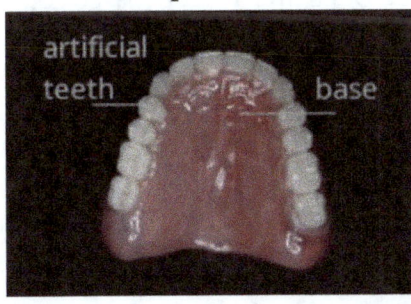
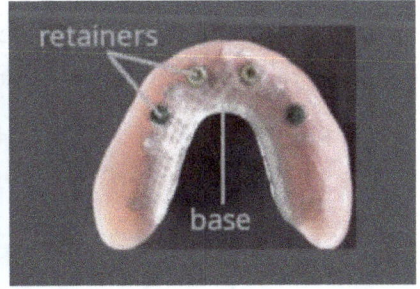

The base of the denture

The denture's base will cover your gum area and the soft tissue of your upper palate. The base will create a replica of your gums, eventually used to craft your custom denture.

Most often, the base of your denture is made of acrylic resin colored matched to your gingival tissue. Another variation is when the base is made of dental ceramics; however, this will entail a much higher cost.

When strength is an essential issue, the acrylic base can be metal-reinforced, or, in some cases, the base can be entirely made of metal (base metal, titanium, or even gold alloys).

When an upper restoration is designed, the base can cover the entire palate or only a part, depending on the clinical conditions.

The artificial teeth

The artificial teeth will replace your missing teeth. The artificial teeth are either stock teeth, delivered by manufacturing companies in various shapes, colors, and sizes, or custom-made teeth, individually fabricated at the dental lab.

Like the base, the artificial teeth can be acrylic (most often) or porcelain. Porcelain teeth will ensure a better aesthetic appearance but are more expensive.

Custom-made teeth can be constructed in any shape and size. When stock teeth are used, a **set** of artificial teeth is selected based on the clinical requirements. For example, women have smaller, more rounded teeth, while men have more prominent teeth.

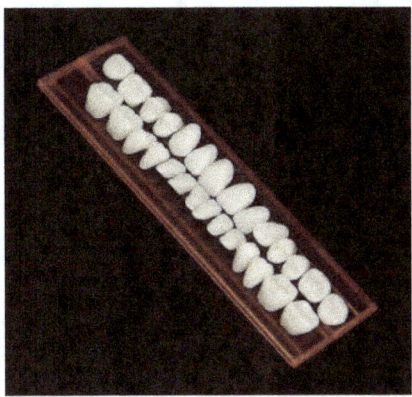

set of stock teeth

Special retainers

As you already know, special retainers hold your denture in place. The retainers have two parts: a *male-adapter* attached to the implant and a *female-adapter* housed in the denture.

Generally, 2 to 8 retainers are utilized for each denture, but the total number will mainly depend on the number and position of dental implants and the overall design of the reconstruction.

The most common types of retainers are the *ball-and-socket style retainer* and the *button-style retainer*. Another variation is the cast metal bar with attachments.

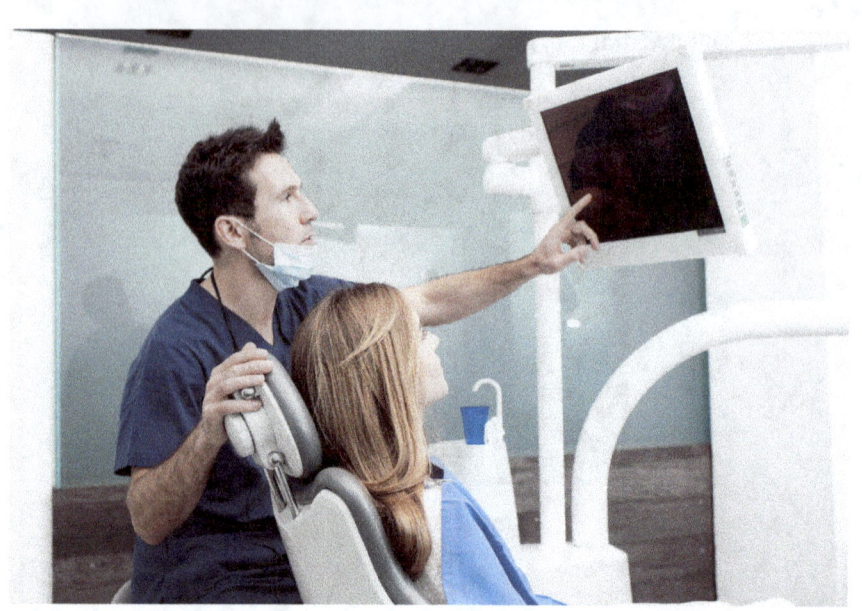

4. Planning For Dental Implants

◆◆◆

In the presence of healthy tissues, well-integrated dental implants with appropriate biomechanical loads can have long-term success rates: 93 to 98 percent for the fixture and 10 to 15 years lifespan for the prosthetic teeth.

For this, proper planning is essential. The medical examination and imaging methods allow the practitioner to devise a treatment plan that should give the implant-supported restoration a long-term success rate.

4.1 Medical Examination

The medical examination will focus on all the essential issues, from general health conditions to local conditions, the assessment of bone support, the soft tissue structure, and the patient's oral hygiene.

The medical examination involves the medical history, an account of the symptoms experienced by the patient, followed by the physical examination.

a. Medical history

During the medical history, your healthcare provider will try to gain helpful information about your general health condition, local conditions, previous surgery, medication, allergies, and others.

This information is vital in planning for implants since some health conditions or drug use may restrict the placement of implants. For example, long-term steroid use, osteoporosis, and other diseases that affect the bones can increase the risk of early failure of implants.

The medical practitioner may ask you specific questions about factors he considers crucial in formulating the diagnosis.

- Identification and demographics - your name, age, height, and weight
- Past medical history - includes major illnesses, any previous surgery/operations, or any current ongoing disease
- Review of systems - systematic questioning about different organ systems
- Family diseases - especially those relevant to the implant treatment
- Childhood diseases relevant to the implant treatment
- Social history - including living arrangements, occupation, marital status, number of children, if you use any drugs (including tobacco, alcohol, or other recreational drugs), oral hygiene status, if you had any recent foreign travel, and exposure to various environmental pathogens.

Patients with poor oral hygiene, heavy smokers, and diabetics are all at greater risk for a variant of inflammatory disease that affects implants called *peri-implantitis*, increasing the chance of long-term failures.

- Regular and acute medications - include those prescribed by doctors and others obtained over-the-counter or alternative medicine.

For example, the use of bone-building drugs, like bisphosphonate drugs, requires special consideration with implants.

- Allergies - to medications, food, latex, and other environmental factors

History-talking may also be available in a printed set of questions you must fill in.

b. Physical examination

During the physical examination, the practitioner carefully investigates your entire oral cavity, focusing on the area needing the implant reconstruction. Specific methods are used: inspection (or visual examination), palpation, and percussion with the help of the examination tools.

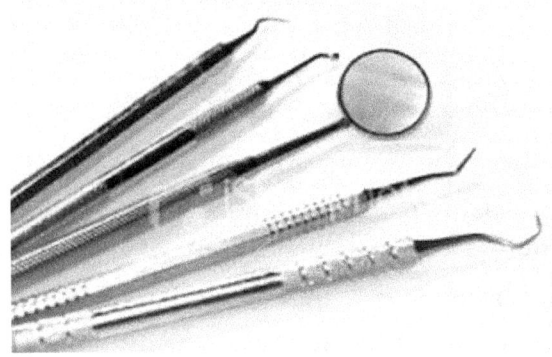

dental examination tools

All key aspects are examined. Additional information will be gathered after the dental radiography and CT scan.

• *Examining the remaining teeth*

Your medical practitioner thoroughly examines your remaining teeth for issues like cavities, erosion, abrasion, color changes, or other pathological conditions. X-rays might be necessary to identify if certain teeth require endodontic treatment.

In some cases, teeth might display significant damage or chronic infections. Based on this, your dentist might opt to extract specific teeth, while others may require endodontic therapy.

Prior to starting the implant procedure, all remaining teeth must receive appropriate treatment.

• Examining the bone support

For an implant to osseointegrate, it needs to be surrounded by a healthy quantity of bone. Therefore, the bone will have to achieve an adequate width and height.

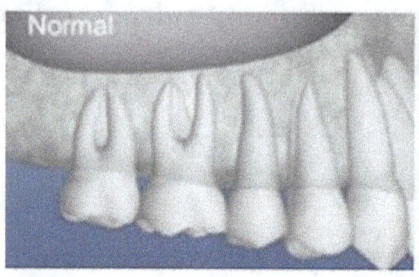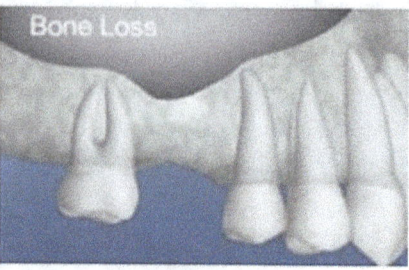

Additional information about the quality and quantity of available bone is gathered after the imaging methods: dental radiography and CT scan.

When the bone is deficient, the surgeon must reconstruct it (either before or during implant placement) using various bone grafting techniques. We'll talk about bone grafting techniques in the next chapter.

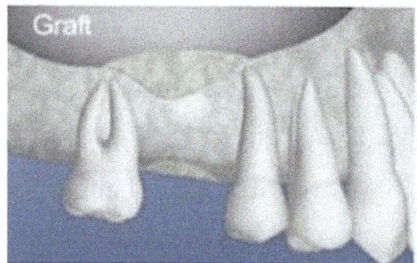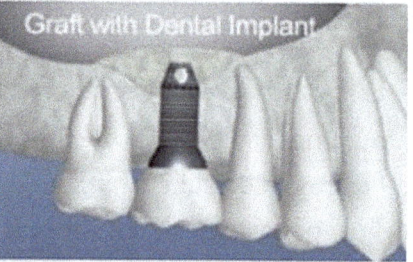

• Examining the occlusion or bite

The long-term success of implants is determined, in part, by the forces they have to support.

Biomechanical forces created during chewing can be significant. Concentrated forces can result in fracture of the bridgework, implant components, or loss of bone adjacent to the implant.

Therefore, the position of dental implants will be selected so that implants distribute forces evenly across the prosthetics they support.

Moreover, an over-eruption (caused by teeth migration) may prevent the proper placement of dental implants and the accurate construction of the prosthetic device because of the lack of space.

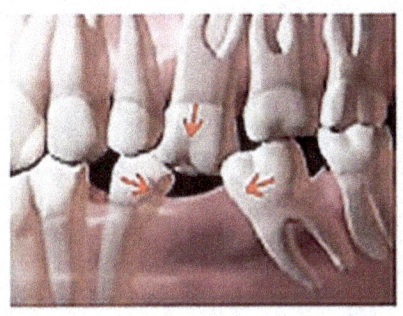

teeth migration may prevent
the proper placement of dental implants

Other conditions, like people who grind their teeth, also increase the force on implants and the likelihood of failures. It is advisable to treat all these conditions before the placement of dental implants.

• Examining the gums and soft tissue support

For optimum success rates, an implant needs to have a thick, healthy soft tissue (gingiva) envelope around it. Soft tissue is sometimes deficient, so the surgeon must reconstruct it.

This procedure is called soft tissue reconstruction; you can read about it in the "Adjunctive Procedures" chapter.

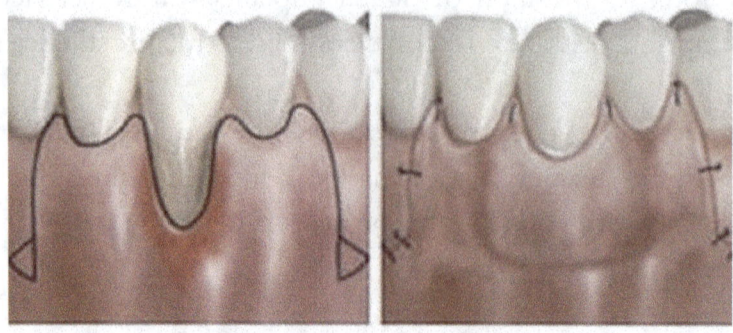

soft tissue reconstruction

Various conditions that affect the oral mucosa may temporarily prevent the placement of dental implants. These conditions will be addressed before the surgical procedure.

• Examining the oral hygiene

Proper and thorough oral hygiene is a prerequisite for successful dental implant rehabilitation. Poor oral hygiene dramatically increases the risk of failure.

Therefore, your dentist or hygienist must help you learn good oral hygiene techniques and point out areas of your mouth that may require extra attention during brushing and flossing.

• Examining the existing restorations

Some of your existing restorations (such as crowns or dental bridges) may need replacement. If this is the case, the quality of the abutment teeth is assessed after their removal. The treatment plan will consider restoring these areas as well.

Every dental practitioner will conduct the medical examination in their own, proven way. The steps described above are only meant to give you a general idea about the process to better understand the importance of proper planning for long-term implant success.

74

4.2 Imaging Methods

When planning for dental implants, imaging methods like dental X-rays, CT scans, or others can significantly help. Imaging methods will give precise information unavailable at the medical examination.

This information is invaluable for an accurate treatment plan.

a. Dental X-ray

Dental X-rays are still the standard way to get an image of the mouth structures prior to placing dental implants. Various views are available:

• *Periapical view*

The periapical view allows the dentist to see both the tooth and the surrounding bone. One or two teeth may be visualized on a single view. It helps diagnose various periapical infections or some bone diseases.

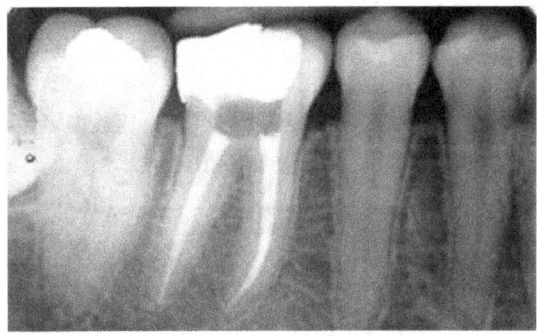

periapical view

The view is also indispensable in assessing the level of osseointegration or bone loss around a dental implant.

Periapical radiographs are often used to determine the need for endodontic therapy and to visualize the successful progression of endodontic therapy once it is initiated.

• Panoramic films

Panoramic films are most often used by dentists when planning for dental implants. Panoramic films are extra-oral films that show all of the teeth as well as the maxillary and mandibular bones.

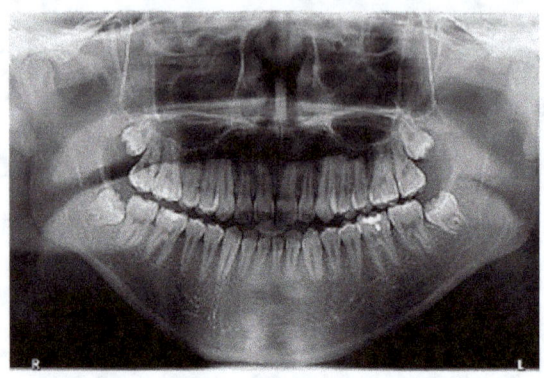

panoramic X-ray

Panoramic films give the practitioner an overall view of the clinical situation, revealing evidence of bone disease, fractures, or other abnormal changes.

• Skull radiography

A skull X-ray is a picture of the bones surrounding the brain, including the facial bones, the nose, and the sinuses.

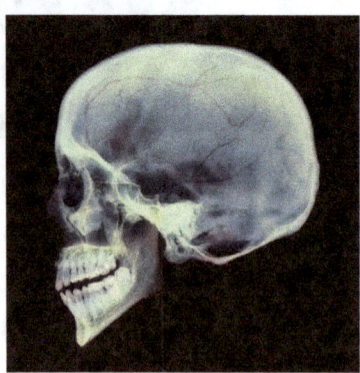

skull radiography

76

Various abnormal conditions may be diagnosed: fractures, tumors, erosions, or decalcifications of the bone.

• Sinus radiography

The sinus view can reveal the position and look of the maxillary sinuses. Because implants are not allowed to penetrate the sinuses, this view might be of great help.

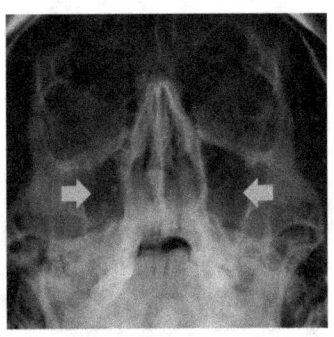

sinus X-ray

Because computed tomography (CT) shows a much clearer picture of the sinuses and surrounding structures, the use of standard sinus X-rays has declined.

What important information can an X-ray bring?

Dental X-rays are essentially like a blueprint for the practitioner, showing whether additional procedures are required to make the implants viable, how large the implants need to be, or where the implants can be placed.

Many important details are available on X-rays:

☐ The quality and quantity (height and width) of available bone

☐ The size and position of critical anatomical structures that might interfere with the dental implants, such as the maxillary sinus or the inferior alveolar nerve in the mandible.

- ☐ Possible infections of the adjacent teeth or the alveolar bone
- ☐ The exact position of the remaining natural teeth

b. CT scan

A computed tomography (CT) scan is an imaging method that uses X-rays to create pictures of cross-sections of the body.

A CT scan provides three-dimensional images of high quality and extreme complexity. CT scanning software is becoming a viable tool in diagnosing dental implant position and placement.

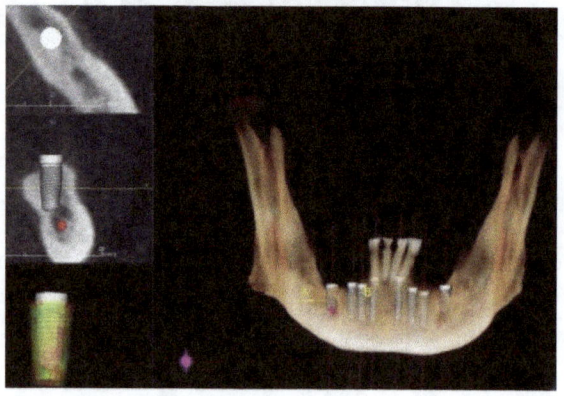

CT scan

The CT scanning software allows the dentist to determine if bone quantity and quality exist and can be used to virtually place dental implants using the computer program before any surgical intervention.

Thus, it eliminates the possible manual placement errors and matches planning to prosthetic requirements.

Besides that, other information is still available on a CT scan: bone infections, possible tumors, blood vessels, and the position of important anatomical structures; the use of CT scanning in complex cases helps the surgeon identify and avoid vital structures such as the inferior alveolar nerve and the sinus.

c. Cone beam computed tomography (CBCT)

A CBCT is a compact, faster, and safer version of the regular CT. Through the use of a cone-shaped X-ray beam, the size of the scanner, radiation dosage, and time needed for scanning are all dramatically reduced.

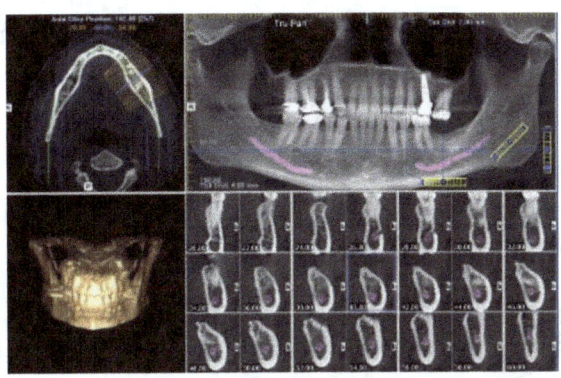

CBCT with more windows

The CBCT produces 3D types images that let the dentist look at mouth structures from different vantage points; it can show the width of mouth structures in addition to their height.

It can also reveal things like cysts and impacted teeth, as well as nerves and arteries that might make the implantation more challenging.

Other imaging methods are available, like an ultrasound or magnetic resonance imaging (MRI) scan. These do not use radiation.

What is *Magnetic Resonance Imaging (MRI)*?

> • **Magnetic Resonance Imaging (MRI) is a medical imaging technique that uses a magnetic field and computer-generated radio waves to create detailed images of the organs and tissues in your body.**

4.3 Treatment Plan

Planning for dental implants is probably the most crucial step of the entire treatment. Depending on the case's complexity, several medical professionals may be involved in this stage.

- *Oral surgeon* - a specialized practitioner who will place the implants inside the jawbone and perform any additional surgical procedures
- *Prosthodontist* - the physician in charge of the prosthetic phase and the general design of the prosthetic restoration
- *Gnatologyst* - in charge of creating a functional occlusion to help distribute the chewing forces evenly across the implant-supported reconstruction
- *Dental technician* - usually with specific training in the field of implantology
- *Physicians of other specialties*

What is *Functional Occlusion*?

- **Functional occlusion, also known as functional bite, is when the teeth of the lower and upper jaws come together in a functional relationship, with the chewing forces distributed evenly across all teeth.**

Creating a functional occlusion is essential for the long-term success of dental implants.

Modern computer software is also available for highly accurate planning.

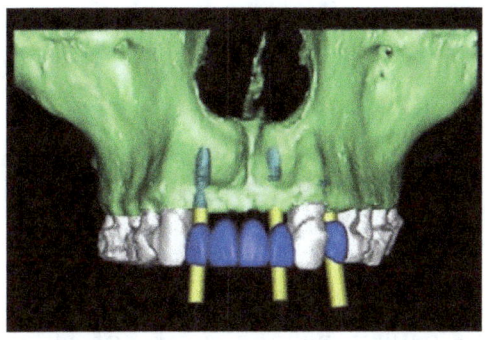

3D dental implant computer planning

An accurate treatment plan will positively impact the implant fixtures' success rate and the prosthetic device's lifespan.

When the treatment plan is designed, all the information gathered during the medical examination and the imaging methods will come together. Moreover, other important factors will have to be considered:

• the dental clinic's facilities and technological equipment: some implant designs need cutting-edge technology that might not be available in every location

• patient preferences for a particular type of restoration; for example, some people prefer to have fixed (permanent) crowns and bridgework instead of removable ones

• patient's financial situation; sometimes, patients cannot afford a particular solution

• available time; many times, an implant restoration needs more time to be completed (up to 6 months), and patients should be available for a various number of appointments

• medical practitioners preferences: most practitioners will opt for proven therapeutic solutions that were successful on other patients treated in the past

• other factors may also be involved; remember that the available therapeutic solutions may be very different depending on the geographic area

What are the main steps in devising the treatment plan?

The treatment plan will address all essential issues. Once completed, the patient will be aware of all the procedures required to finalize the implant-supported restoration.
Several steps might be involved:

a. General considerations

As we pointed out in the previous chapter, some severe general health conditions absolutely preclude placing implants, while other situations are evaluated on a case-by-case basis.
In such situations, your doctor may recommend an appointment to a specialist physician (depending on the medical condition, this may be a cardiologist, an oncologist, or another specialized health care provider).

b. The treatment of all existing mouth conditions

Before any surgical procedure, all structures inside the mouth cavity should be adequately treated.
   • The treatment of teeth decays
   • The treatment of gingivitis, periodontal disease, and any other soft tissue conditions
   • Endodontic therapy for teeth with chronic infections
   • Professional dental cleaning and scaling
   • Removal of the teeth that can no longer be treated

c. Selecting the type of implant-supported prosthesis

The final prosthetic can be either fixed, where a person cannot remove the teeth from their mouth, or removable, where they can remove the prosthetic.

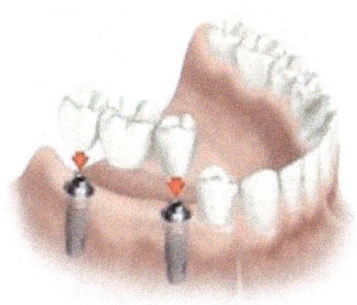 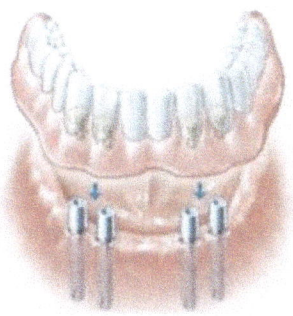

implant-supported bridge   *implant-supported denture*

For example, an implant-supported bridge is a fixed restoration, while an implant-supported denture should be removed daily for cleaning.

Where the prosthetic is fixed, the dental crown or bridge is attached to the abutments with either lag screws or cement. Where the prosthetic is removable, a corresponding adapter is placed in the prosthetic so that the two pieces can be secured together.

d. Selecting the number of implants and the type and position of each dental implant

Planning the position and number of implants is key to the long-term health of the prosthetic since biomechanical forces created during chewing can be significant.

I. Number

The number of implants directly depends on the type of prosthetic restoration. Normally, a removable denture needs fewer supporting implants than a fixed denture (although this is not a general rule).

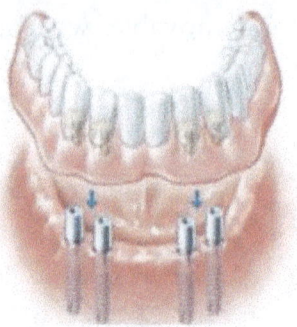

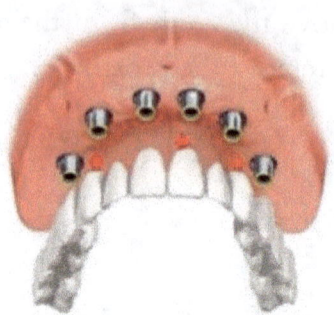

removable denture can be supported by four implants

a fixed denture needs more supporting implants

II. Position

Dental implants have no periodontal ligament; hence, there is no sensation of pressure when biting. Consequently, the forces created are higher.

To offset this, the location of implants must distribute forces evenly across the prosthetics they support. Concentrated forces can result in fracture of the bridgework, implant components, or loss of bone adjacent to the implants.

Implants' ultimate location is based on both biological (bone type, vital structures, health) and mechanical factors. Implants placed in thicker, stronger bone (e.g., the front part of the bottom jaw) have lower failure rates than implants placed in lower-density bone (such as the back part of the upper jaw).

When a more exacting plan is needed, the dentist can make an acrylic or plastic guide called a guidance stent. The guidance stent is manufactured prior to surgery and guides the optimal positioning of the implants.

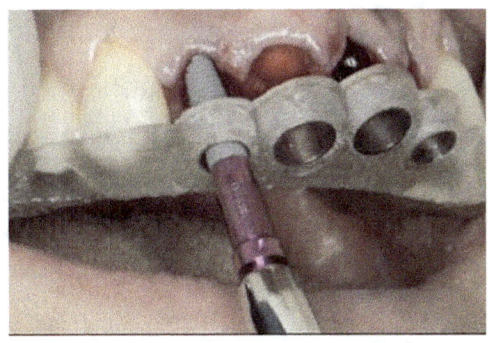

guidance stent during surgery

The stent can be made following the computerized planning of a case from the CT scan.

III. Type

Dental implants and abutments come in a wide range of sizes and shapes. The practitioner will select the implants and the abutments that best fit the clinical application.

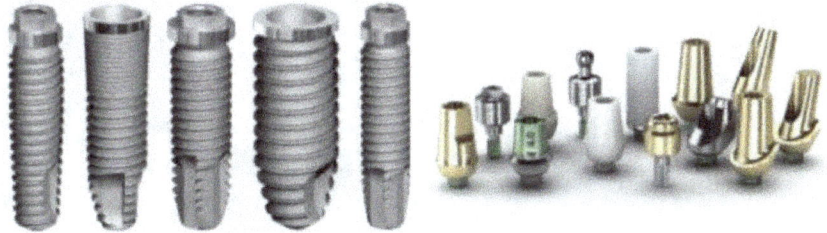

dental implants of various sizes   *implant abutments of multiple types*

Most often, larger implants (and artificial abutments) are selected for the back part of the mouth due to the increased chewing forces (although this is not a general rule).

The length and diameter of dental implants ultimately depend on the bone structure and the type of prosthesis that is planned.

e. Planning the adjunctive surgical procedures

When the bone's size or structure is insufficient to support the implants, additional surgical procedures such as bone grafts or sinus lifts are planned to increase the amount of bone.

Other techniques aim to recreate the soft tissues surrounding the implants or to reposition anatomical structures that might interfere with the dental implants (e.g., soft tissue reconstruction, alveolar nerve repositioning, sinus lift).

Generally, the adjunctive procedures are performed before the implant positioning (although, in some situations, these can be performed during implant placement).

Lastly, every procedure is precisely scheduled, and all essential details are clarified.

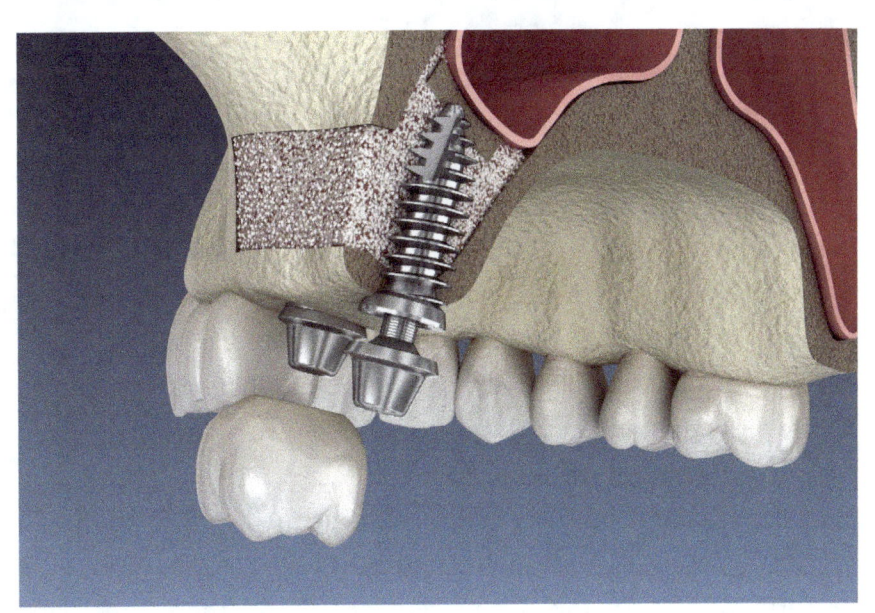

5. Adjunctive Surgical Procedures

◆◆◆

For an implant to osseointegrate, it needs to be surrounded by a healthy quantity of bone. Moreover, a band of strong, attached gingiva is required to keep the implant healthy in the long term. When bone or soft tissue is deficient, adjunctive surgical procedures are performed to increase the amount of bone or reconstruct the soft tissues surrounding the implant.

Some clinical situations will not require adjunctive procedures. However, when the case calls for such procedures, they are essential for long-term success.

Usually, adjunctive procedures are performed before the main implant procedure, although in some situations, these may be performed during implant placement. While there are many types of adjunctive procedures, these are the most common:

- **Sinus lift** - is a standard surgical procedure that aims to provide sufficient bone under the maxillary (upper jaw) sinus for dental implant placement.

- **Bone grafting** - is a surgical procedure that replaces missing bone with material from the patient's own body, an artificial, synthetic, or natural substitute.

In the case of dental implants, bone grafting is used to increase the amount of bone in the jaw to help with the best positioning of dental implants.

- **Soft tissue reconstruction (or gum graft)** - is a generic name for any of a number of surgical procedures whose combined aim is to cover an area of exposed tooth root surface or dental implant with grafted oral tissue.

- **Alveolar nerve repositioning** - is a surgical procedure whereby the course of the inferior alveolar nerve is redirected to allow the placement of dental implants in a mandible with extensive resorption of the posterior ridge.

In the next subchapters, we will detail the first three procedures, which are the most often used.

5.1 Sinus Lift

Sinus lift (also termed sinus floor augmentation, sinus graft, or sinus procedure) is a surgical procedure that aims to increase the amount of bone in the posterior maxilla (upper jaw bone) in the area of premolar and molar teeth by sacrificing some of the volume of the maxillary sinus.

The two maxillary sinuses are tiny air-filled holes located below the cheeks, above the back teeth (molar and premolars), and on the sides of the nose.

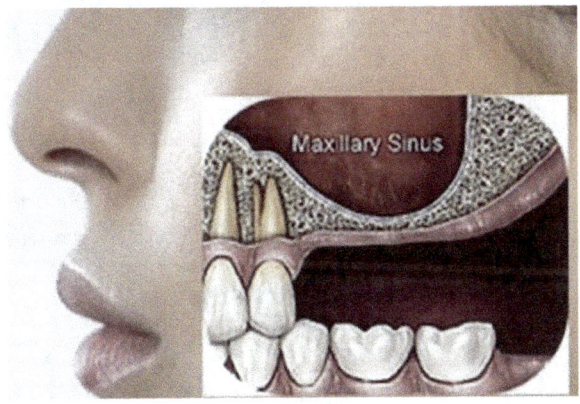

While there may be a number of reasons for wanting a greater volume of bone in the posterior maxilla, the most common reason in contemporary dental treatment planning is to prepare the site for the future placement of dental implants.

What may cause the lowering of the sinuses?

Several factors may cause the lowering of the sinuses:

1. Long-term tooth loss without the required treatment

When a natural tooth is lost due to dental decay, periodontal disease, or dental trauma, the alveolar process begins to remodel.

The toothless area (termed edentulous ridge) will usually lose both height and width over time. Furthermore, the level of the maxillary sinus floor gradually becomes lower.

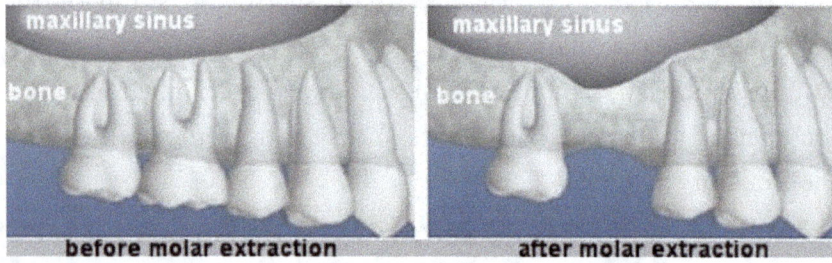

In advanced stages of periodontal disease, bone loss is typically higher.

Overall, this leads to a loss of bone volume that is available for implantation of dental implants, which rely on osseointegration.

2. Inflammation of the maxillary sinuses

Sometimes, an inflammatory condition of the maxillary sinuses (called *sinusitis*) may lead to bone resorption and the lowering of the sinus floor.

3. Congenital disorders

Some patients may have the maxillary sinuses enlarged from birth due to a genetic defect.

4. Other causes

Other causes can include enhanced bone resorption at this level, missing teeth due to genetics or birth defects, or trauma.

Surgical procedure

Sinus augmentation (sinus lift) is performed when the floor of the sinus is too close to an area where dental implants are to be placed.

This procedure ensures a secure place for the implants while protecting the sinus.

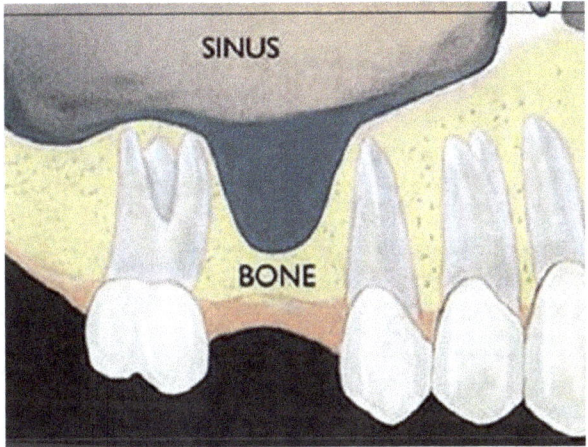

a clinical situation where sinus lift is indicated

Preparation

Prior to undergoing sinus augmentation, diagnostics are run to determine the health of the patient's sinuses, general health, and other local conditions.

Panoramic radiographs are taken to map out the patient's upper jaw and sinuses. CT scan is taken to measure the sinus's height and width and to rule out any sinus disease or pathology.

Technique

All procedures involve bone grafting, which adds bone volume to the sinus floor. Various materials may be utilized:

- *autogenous bone*: a bone graft taken from elsewhere on the individual's body, e.g., the back of the head, iliac crest, etc
- *biomaterials*: artificial substances that replace human bone, e.g., calcium sulfate, hydroxyapatite

Operation explained

Typically, the procedure is performed under general anesthesia.

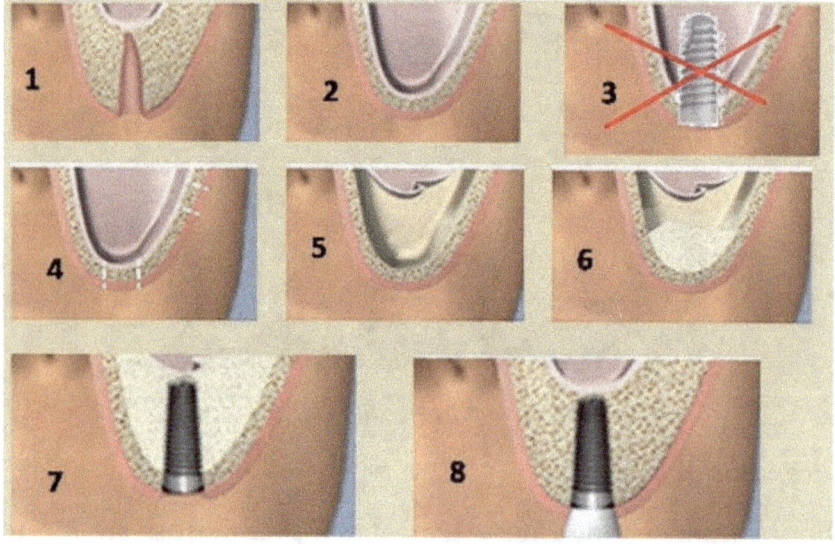

1. Tooth loss leads to bone loss.

2. Over time, the sinus will expand into the area previously occupied by bone and teeth.

3. If a dental implant is placed into inadequate bone, it will move, shift, and eventually fail.

4. The sinus lift procedure begins with a temporary opening in one of the two possible areas.

5. With a surgical instrument, the *sinus membrane* is carefully lifted to its previous position, providing clearance for the placement of the substitute bone (the bone graft).

6. Adequate bone is placed to provide support for the dental implant.

7. Over time, the implant and substitute bone will heal, creating a solid bond.

8. The implant-supported crown has a stable foundation.

Now, let's see how the maxillary sinus looks before and after the procedure:

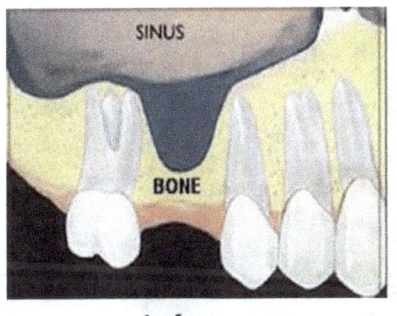
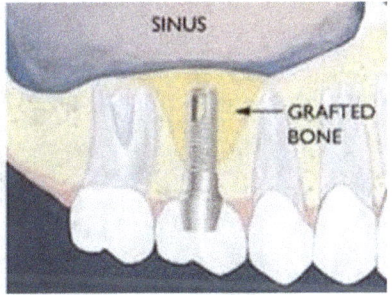

before   *after*

Sinus lift complications

A major risk of a sinus augmentation is that the sinus membrane could be pierced or ripped (most often during step 5). Should this occur, the therapeutic remedies include stitching the tear or placing a patch over it.

In some cases, the surgery is stopped altogether, and the tear is given time to heal. The sinus membrane often grows back thicker and more robust, making success more likely on the second operation.

Other risks include infection, inflammation, hematoma, pain, graft failure, or sinusitis.

However, the overall success rate of a proper sinus lift procedure is excellent (95 to 97%).

5.2 Bone Grafting

Bone grafting is a surgical procedure that replaces missing bone to repair bone fractures that are extremely complex or increase the amount of bone in a particular site for various reasons.

In dental implantology, bone grafting is necessary when there is **a** lack of bone. For an implant to osseointegrate, it needs to be surrounded by a healthy quantity of bone.

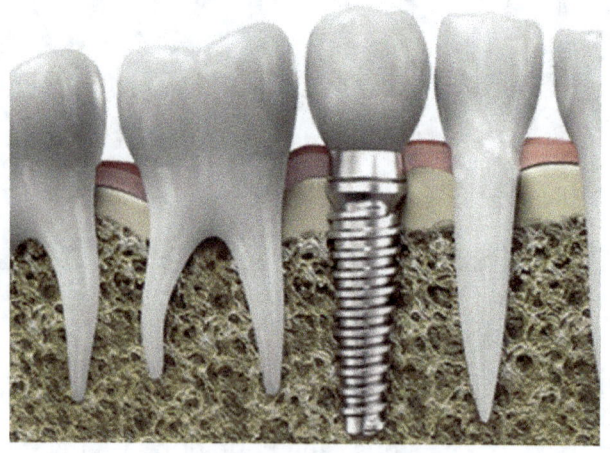

dental implant surrounded
by healthy bone tissue

While there are always new implant types and techniques to allow compromise, a general treatment goal is to have a minimum of **10 mm in bone height and 6 mm in width.**

Bone loss causes

Bone is lost through a biological process called *bone resorption*. Many reasons can cause excessive bone loss:

• Long-term teeth loss

When natural teeth are lost, the sites that remain after the extractions begin a remodeling process. Over time, the toothless areas will gradually lose height and width.

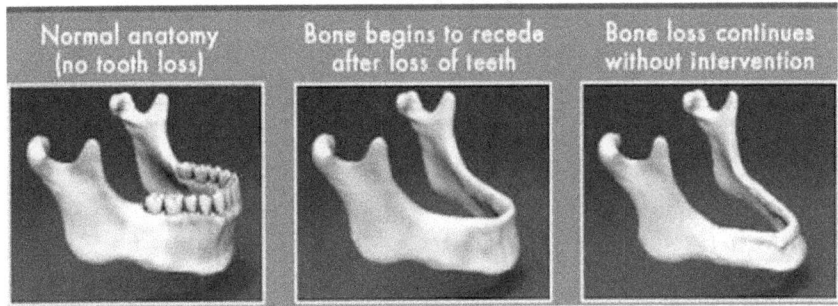

mandible bone recession after teeth loss

The bone resorption process occurs when toothless areas remain unrestored. The amount of bone loss is significantly reduced when a dental prosthesis is designed to restore the toothless gap, especially if dental implants support it.

• Periodontal disease

Periodontitis (or advanced periodontal disease) is a destructive disease involving a significant resorption of the alveolar bone tissue. If left untreated, it can lead to the loosening and subsequent loss of teeth.

Progression of Bacteria and Periodontitis

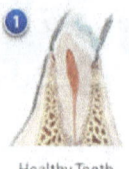 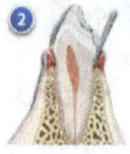 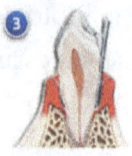 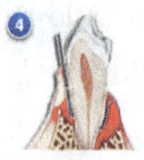

| Healthy Teeth and Gums | **Stage 1** Gingivitis | **Stage 2** Gum Recession & Moderate Periodontitis | **Stage 3** Advanced Periodontal Disease & Bone Loss |

progression of periodontal disease

When teeth are lost through periodontal disease, the bone left behind has already diminished significantly in height and width. An implant procedure in these circumstances is highly challenging.

• Bone disease

Various bone diseases, such as bone infections, osteoporosis, fractures, tumors, or following surgical interventions or radiation therapy, can stimulate the process of bone resorption, which results in a high amount of bone loss.

Surgical procedure

Various bone grafting techniques have been developed to achieve adequate bone width and height. Typically, the bone defects are filled with grafting materials, which are then covered with a *semi*-permeable membrane.

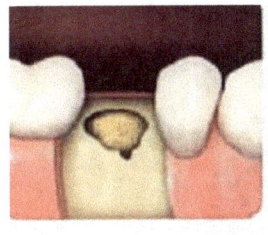
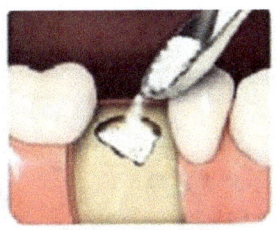
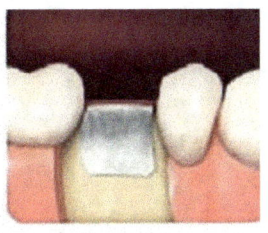

| bone defect | bone defect is filled with grafting materials | finally, all is covered with a membrane |

During the healing phase, natural bone replaces the graft, forming a new bony base for the implant and adding volume to the bone. The process is called *guided bone regeneration (GBR)*.

Grafting materials

There are two types of grafting materials:

- **Autograft**: natural bone harvested from large body sources, such as the iliac crest, the back of the head, or others.
- **Allograft**: artificial substances that replace human bone and stimulate natural bone formation, such as calcium sulfate or hydroxyapatite.

Techniques

Three standard procedures involve bone graft: sinus lift (described in the previous subchapter), lateral alveolar augmentation, and vertical alveolar augmentation.

• Lateral alveolar augmentation

Lateral alveolar augmentation is the increase in the width of a site. The procedure may be performed both at the upper and lower jawbones.

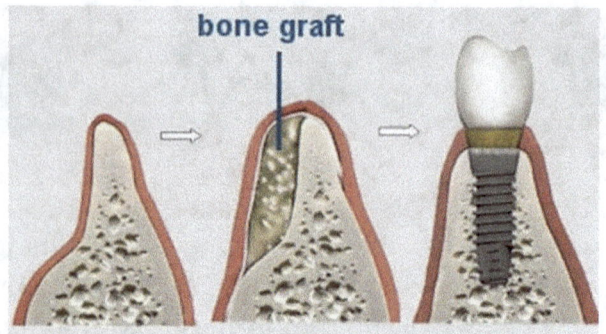

Whenever the bone width is insufficient, it is advisable to resort to these procedures, which are relatively simple, painless, and with an excellent success rate.

• Vertical alveolar augmentation

Vertical alveolar augmentation is the increase in the height of a site. The procedure is crucial if bone height is insufficient; dental implants placed in deficient bone have a high risk of failure.

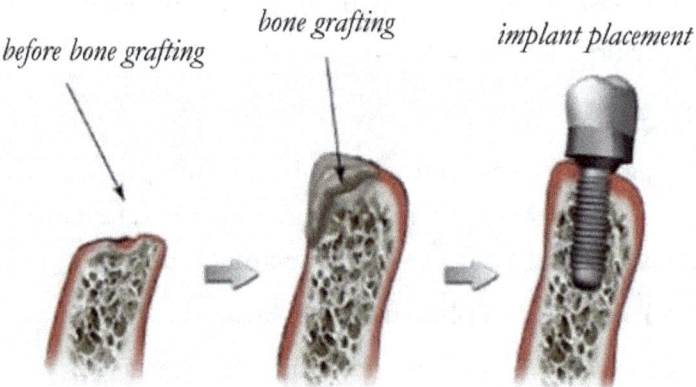

• Other techniques

Other, more complex procedures also exist for sizable bone defects. These are performed under general anesthesia by the oral surgeon.

For example, the mobilization (or repositioning) of the inferior alveolar nerve (located inside the mandible) is indicated when the nerve has an abnormal position that does not allow proper placement of the implant fixtures.

The final decision about which bone grafting technique will be performed is based on assessing the degree of vertical and horizontal bone loss: mild, moderate, or severe.

5.3 Soft Tissue Reconstruction

Soft tissue reconstruction (also called gum graft or gingival graft) is a generic name for any of a number of surgical procedures whose combined aim is to cover an area of exposed tooth root surface or dental implant with grafted oral tissue.

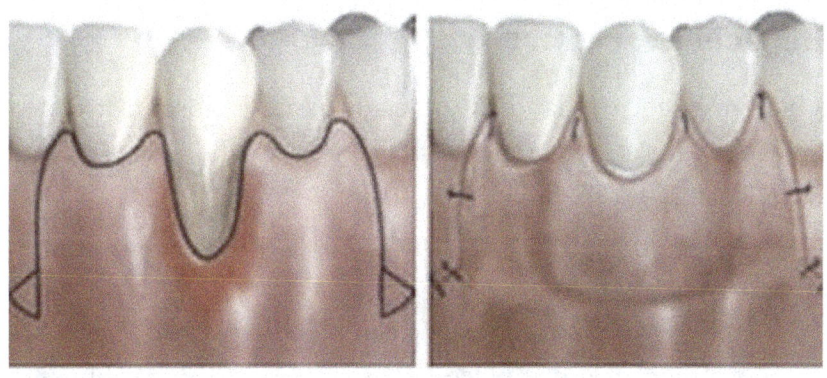

an example of a gum graft to cover
an area of exposed tooth root

The normal gingiva

The healthy gum (or gingiva) surrounding a tooth has a 2-3 mm band of bright pink, very strong attached mucosa (marked with **a**, image below), then a darker, more extensive area of unattached mucosa that folds into the cheeks (marked with **b**, image bellow).

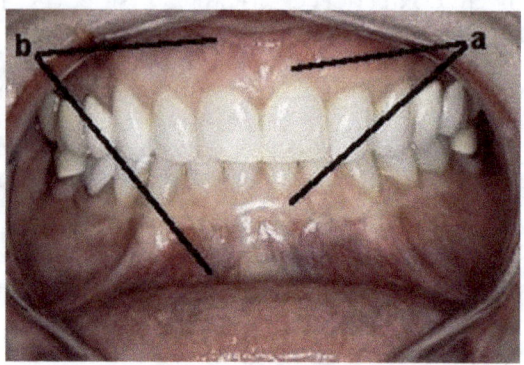

When replacing a tooth with an implant, a band of strong, attached gingiva is needed to keep the implant healthy in the long term. This is especially important with implants because the blood supply is more precarious in the soft tissues surrounding an implant.

Surgical procedure

When an adequate band of attached tissue is absent, it can be recreated with a soft tissue graft. Various methods can be used to transplant soft tissue:

• A roll of tissue adjacent to an implant can be moved towards the area

• Gingiva from the palate can be transplanted

• When a larger piece of tissue is needed, a "finger of tissue" based on a blood vessel in the palate can be repositioned to the area

Example

Gingival grafting to increase the zone of attached gum tissue around a dental implant:

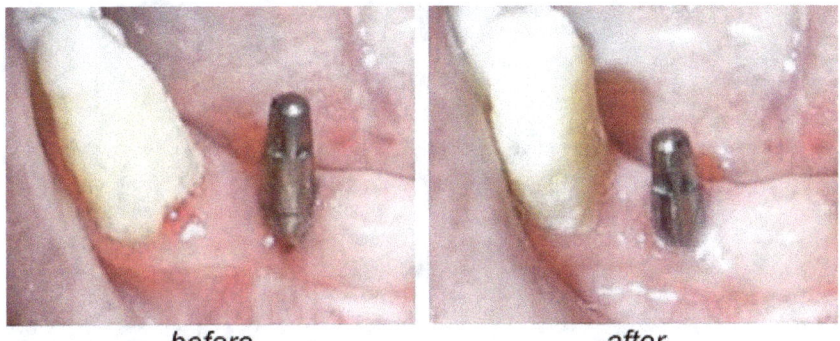

before   *after*

Additionally, for an implant to look aesthetic, a band of full, plump gingiva is needed to fill in the space on either side of the implant.

The most common soft tissue complication is called a *black-triangle*, where the papilla (the small triangular piece of tissue between two teeth) shrinks back and leaves a triangular void between the implant crown and the adjacent teeth.

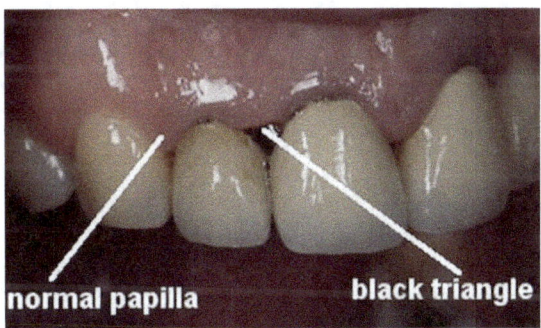

Generally, after the adjunctive surgical procedures are completed, a healing time is required before the implant placement can actually begin. The amount of healing time may vary depending on the type of procedures that were performed.

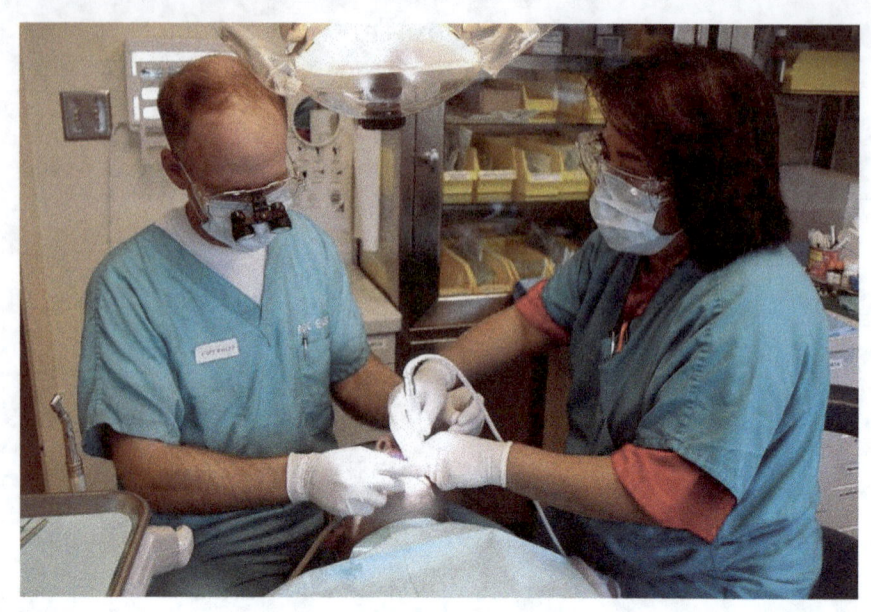

6. Dental Implant Procedure

❖❖❖

Before we start with the dental implant procedure, some important considerations regarding the timing of this process.

When we plan to replace one or several teeth with dental implants, there are different approaches to the placement of dental implants after tooth extraction:

• Immediate post-extraction implant placement

An increasingly common strategy to preserve bone and reduce treatment time includes the placement of a dental implant into a recent extraction site.

On the one hand, it shortens treatment time and can improve aesthetics because the soft tissue envelope is preserved.

On the other hand, implants may have a slightly higher initial failure rate. We will have more on the subject when we discuss the *Same-day dental implants*.

• Delayed immediate post-extraction implant placement

The implant is placed two weeks to three months after the tooth extraction. The procedure requires bone grafting to create a bony base for the implant.

• Late implantation

The surgery is performed three months or more after tooth extraction. It is the most prudent approach; during this time, the body will grow new bone inside the alveolar socket, where the tooth was formerly held.

6.1 Dental Implant Surgery

The surgical placement of dental implants is a painless procedure that can last a variable time (from 10 min to 2 hours) depending on how many implants are inserted.

The dental implant procedure is normally performed by the oral surgeon or another specialized physician under *local anesthesia*. However, in some cases, *general anesthesia* can also be used.

Surgery technique

Most implant systems have five basic steps for the placement of each implant.

1. Soft tissue reflection

This step aims to expose the bone in the area where the implant is placed. An incision is made over the crest of the bone, splitting the soft tissue.

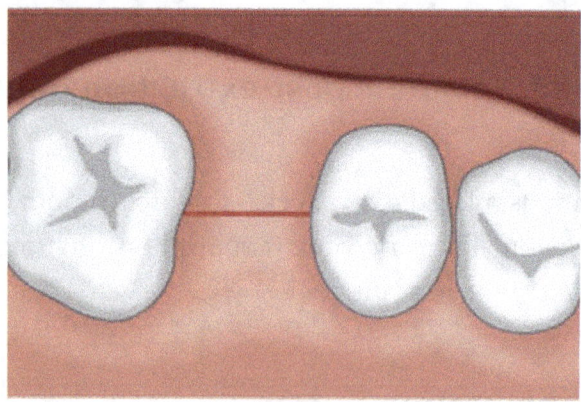

incision

The edges of tissue, each referred to as a *flap*, are pushed back to expose the bone.

Flapless surgery is an alternate technique where a small punch of tissue (the diameter of the implant) is removed for implant placement rather than raising flaps.

2. Drilling

For this operation, the oral surgeon makes use of specific titanium drills. A cooling saline or water spray keeps the temperature low to prevent bone damage caused by overheating.

• The surgeon may use a *guidance stent* to guide the optimal positioning of the implants.

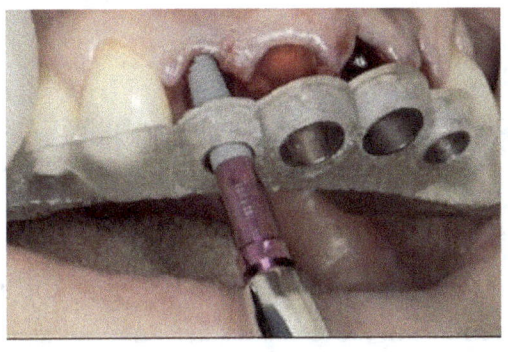

guidance stent

• Pilot holes are placed with precision drills at highly regulated speeds to prevent burning or pressure necrosis of the bone.

• The pilot holes are expanded using progressively wider drills. Three to seven successive drilling steps may be needed depending on implant width and length.

• The last drill used matches implant dimensions (width and length)

3. Placement of the implants

The implant is screwed into place at a precise torque so as not to overload the surrounding bone (which may cause osteonecrosis and implant failure). A specific screw-key is utilized for the operation.

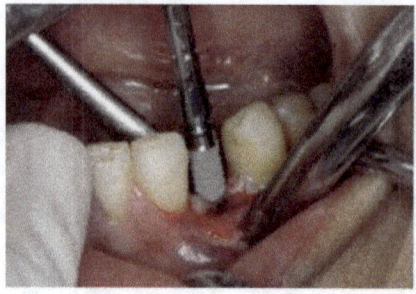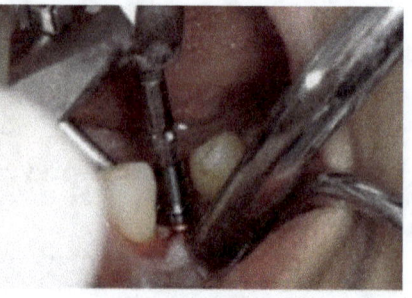

placement of the implant phase 1   *placement of the implant phase 2*

4. Soft tissue adaptation

After the implant placement, a specific healing device is screwed into the implant. There are two possible alternatives:

• Healing abutment

The healing abutment passes through the mucosa and the surrounding soft tissues are adapted around it.

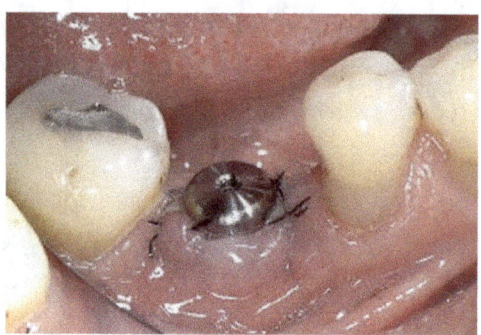

healing abutment

• Cover screw

The cover screw is flush with the surface of the dental implant and is designed to be entirely covered by mucosa. A second procedure would then be required to uncover the implant at a later date (two-stage procedure).

The choice of one or two-stage procedure centers on how best to reconstruct the soft tissues around lost teeth.

The gingiva is adapted around the entire implant to provide a thick band of healthy tissue around the healing abutment.

When a cover screw is used, the implant is "buried" and the tissue is closed to cover it completely.

5. Temporary restoration

When the procedure is completed, the practitioner will construct a temporary restoration that will replace the missing teeth during the biological process of osseointegration (which usually takes 3 to 6 months).

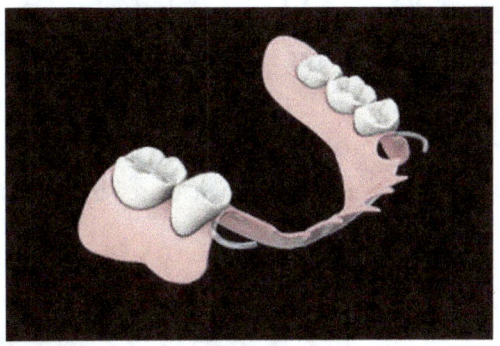

commonly, a temporary partial denture
will replace the missing teeth

After the operation

After the surgical procedure, the oral surgeon may prescribe pain relievers, anti-inflammatory medication, and antibiotics.

It is advisable to protect the areas where the procedure was performed in the early days after surgery. Proper and thorough oral hygiene is essential.

Most often, there are no significant side effects. Bruising and swelling of the gums and face, pain, and minor bleeding are not uncommon - and do not necessarily indicate that something has gone wrong. However, it is wise to keep the surgeon apprised of those symptoms.

Sutures are usually removed after 7-10 days. During this appointment, the doctor will also assess the healing process.

Placement of dental implants is a surgical procedure and carries the normal risks of surgery. We will discuss these risks later.

6.2 Healing And Osseointegration

For an implant to become permanently stable, the body must grow bone to the surface of the implant. This process is called *osseointegration.*

Osseointegration is defined as the formation of a direct interface between an implant and bone without intervening soft tissue.

Applied to oral implantology, this means that the bone grows right up to the implant surface without an interposed soft tissue layer.

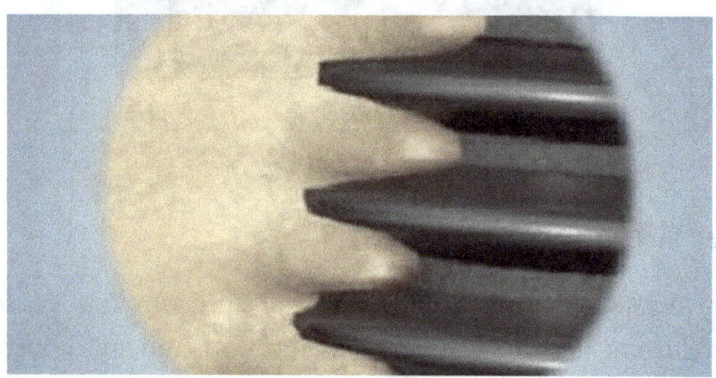

When osseointegration occurs, the implant is tightly held in place by the bone. The process typically takes several weeks or months.

Several factors can influence osseointegration:

• Implant material

For osseointegrated dental implants, metallic, ceramic (zirconia), and polymeric materials, particularly titanium, have been used. Up to this day, titanium is the most favored material due to its remarkable ability to connect its surface with the alveolar bone. However, zirconia dental implants have recently emerged. Even though they are relatively new, there has been a considerable increase in the use of these types of implants.

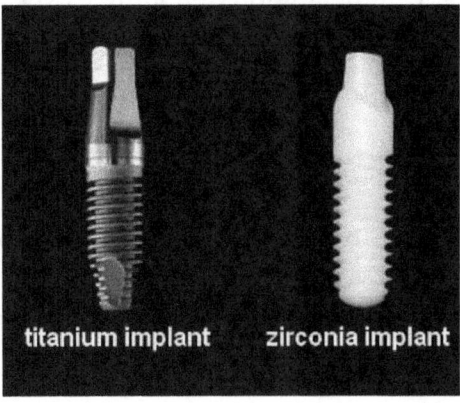

titanium implant   zirconia implant

• Loading time

Loading time refers to the moment when the artificial teeth are attached to the implants.

Refrain from confusing *loading time* with the *timing of implants after teeth extraction*.

The first refers to when the artificial teeth are attached to the implants.

The second refers to when the implants are placed after tooth extraction.

Generally speaking, osseointegration can be damaged by prolonged adverse stimuli and overload, possibly resulting in implant failure. However, there are three valid options for when to attach teeth to dental implants:

• *Immediate loading procedure*

Immediate loading means that the artificial abutments and (sometimes) the prosthetic restoration are attached to the implants during the surgical placement procedure (or immediately after).

This relatively new approach aims to shorten treatment time. Followers suggest that the initial stability of the implant in bone is a more important determinant of the success of implant integration rather than a certain period of healing time.

• *Early loading*

Early loading means that abutments and artificial teeth are attached to the implants one to twelve weeks after surgery.

These two loading methods have certain limitations. Even in the event of early or immediate loading, many practitioners prefer to place temporary restorations for a specific time.

Once the implants have had a chance to heal and have been tested for successful integration, the definitive restoration is manufactured.

• *Delayed loading*

It is the most prudent approach; three to six months of integrating time is allowed before placing the teeth on implants.

Before connecting the artificial abutments, the implants are tested for successful osseointegration.

The fact is that the degree of osseointegration of implants is a matter of time. While the first evidence of integration occurs after a few weeks, the more robust connection is progressively achieved over the following months or years.

As a result, the osseointegration process continues well after the definitive restoration is secured to the implants.

That is one reason why the prosthetic phase requires equal technical expertise: a restoration that overloads one (or more) implants can damage the osseointegration process, which may result in implant failure.

In the following subchapter, we'll explore a relatively new approach where the entire dental implant procedure is performed in a single day.

6.3 Same-Day Dental Implants

Dental implants have many benefits. One of the most important is replacing a broken or damaged tooth in the front area that can no longer be restored.

In this case, an implant crown offers a highly aesthetic and efficient solution as it avoids the need to prepare the adjacent teeth.

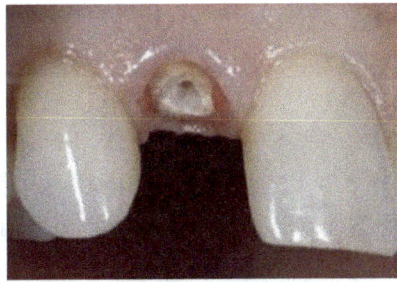

broken front tooth
that can no longer be restored

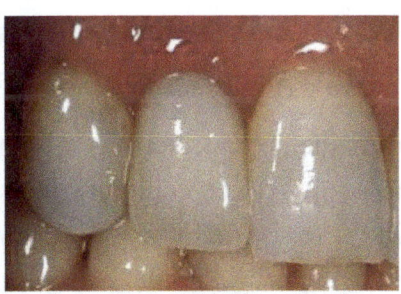

after tooth removal, a dental implant
is placed to restore the gap

However, the traditional procedure can take up to one year as it implies three different steps:

a.   Removal of the existing tooth or root; the extraction socket is left to heal for four to six months before a dental implant is placed. During this period, the body will grow new bone inside the socket.

b.   The implant is surgically inserted into the jaw bone. A variable healing time is required for osseointegration (3 to 6 months). Osseointegration is a biological process where the implant forms an intimate bond to the bone.

c.   After the healing time, a dental crown is attached to the implant.

Teeth in a day: Immediate placement and loading

Patient demand for immediate gratification has increased; as a result, implant dentistry has since responded with immediate implant placement after extraction, followed by immediate loading of the crown.

Immediate loading is becoming far more common: the implant and temporary crown are placed within 48 hours of implant surgery and left in position for the healing period.

Who is a candidate for immediate tooth replacement with implants?

Immediate placement is not appropriate for all patients and cases, and the screening process should be comprehensive.

The ideal candidate is someone who is in good dental and general health. Some factors can also negatively affect dental implants:

- smoking
- any conditions that affect the immune system or reduce the body's ability to heal
- some drugs, such as *bisphosphonates*, as these drugs increase the risk of bone death after surgery
- bruxism or teeth grinding and clenching

Patients who choose this approach must be committed to good oral hygiene. Furthermore, not overloading the implant crown is another factor that needs to be reinforced when loading an implant immediately after placement.

Patients with enough bone quantity and quality are great candidates for immediate placement and loading because of anticipated implant initial stability, assuming they would comply with postoperative instructions.

Procedure steps

There are a number of issues and steps to consider:

1. Consultation and planning

Dental implant surgery has to be meticulously planned; when you opt for immediate implant placement, careful planning and experience are prerequisites for success.

Your dentist will need to know your complete dental and medical history before carrying out various diagnostic tests, such as dental X-rays and a CT scan.

Your clinician will analyze the data from these tests to assess the quality of the bone that will be surrounding the dental implant.

When an implant is placed into a recent extraction site, many doctors prefer to graft bone in the alveolar socket to create a bony base for the implant.

There should also be enough gum tissue to surround the implant and crown, as this will affect aesthetics; the implant-crown should look like it is emerging naturally from the gums. Gingival tissue can be grafted from another site in the mouth if necessary.

At this stage, the dentist will also determine the best position for the implant and choose the correct size.

2. Removing the existing tooth

It is critical that your broken tooth is removed very carefully so that the tooth socket is not damaged.

If any bone from the walls of the socket is damaged or lost, it could lead to unsightly gum recession and a poor prognosis; in this case, many practitioners would prefer to end the procedure (and continue with the traditional approach) rather than risk a poor result.

3. Implant placement

When the same-day dental implant technique is used, your doctor will place the implant fixture in the bone right after the tooth extraction.

It is vital to place the implant in a stable and non-movable place in the bone. This stability is referred to as the primary stability of the implant.

The latest research suggests that the primary stability of the implant in bone is a more critical determinant of the success of implant integration rather than a certain period of healing time.

The tooth socket of an upper front tooth is cone-shaped. To achieve primary stability, the implant has to penetrate the apex of the socket (or the endpoint) and affix into the bone in this area (see image below).

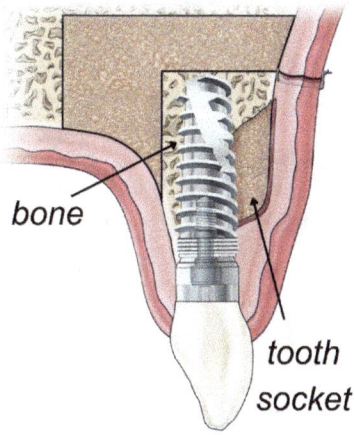

bone

tooth
socket

Additionally, a bone graft can be placed inside the tooth socket. Selecting the right-sized implant and ensuring it is placed in the correct position is essential.

4. Crown placement

The crown will be attached to the implant in one of two ways:

- Directly: the crown and the abutment are one piece, and a lag screw traverses both to secure the one-piece structure to the internal thread on the implant.
- Indirectly: first, the abutment is attached to the implant, and the crown will be cemented to the abutment. In this variation, the abutment can be used to create a change of angulation for the crown to emerge through the gum tissue with a more natural appearance.

Regardless of the variation, the newly attached crown must be free from biting forces, which could displace the implant. The crown is usually a temporary crown made of a composite or acrylic resin, which can easily be modified to ensure that it is both functional and cosmetic.

Once the implant is fully integrated with the bone, the temporary crown can be removed and replaced with a permanent one.

5. Care and maintenance

Immediate implant placement and loading require higher patient compliance. There are three key factors that patients have to consider:

• Overloading

The implant restoration must be manageable as even micro-movement during the first two months of placement can result in non-fusion and failure of the implant to attach to the surrounding bone.

Avoid biting on extremely hard pieces of food, and contact your doctor if you notice any signs of involuntary teeth grinding and clenching.

• Oral hygiene

To prevent infection, taking good care of the area around the implant for the first couple of months after the surgery is critical.

If maintaining this level of care could be a problem, then you should consider traditional dental implants that use a two-stage technique.

• Smoking

You may not be suitable for this type of treatment if you are a heavy smoker and have problems quitting smoking and tobacco products.

Benefits and risks of same-day dental implants

a. Benefits

• *Reduced treatment time*

A traditional implant can take six months to one year to completely restore, considering the tooth removal the starting point.

Same-day implants can replace a front tooth almost immediately.

• *Only one surgical procedure is required*

Tooth removal, implant placement, and crown attachment are all performed during the same visit. Consequently, there is no need to uncover the implant 3-6 months later to attach the abutment and crown.

• *Better aesthetic results are achieved regarding the gum tissue*

With immediate placement and loading, the temporary crown can shape the gum tissue. As a result, the gum tissue matches the permanent crown, and better aesthetic results are achieved.

• *It avoids the need for temporary dentures or the "missing teeth" look*

Since the implant crown is attached in the same procedure, there is no need to wear a removable denture or have gaps in your smile during the healing period.

In the traditional implant procedure, the practitioner will construct a temporary restoration to replace the missing teeth after the implant placement.

b. Risks and drawbacks

• *Even the slightest movement increases the risk of failure*

Same-day implant placement is a very precise technique. The practitioner must take all necessary measures to ensure the implant cannot move while integrating with the bone, especially in the first two months.

• *The technique is only suitable for specific situations*

As mentioned, same-day implants are not appropriate for all patients and cases, and the selection process is an essential step of this treatment.

• *The implant surgeon has to be skilled and experienced*

Same-day implants cannot be performed by anyone. The surgeon must be skillful and experienced enough to place the dental implant accurately to eliminate the risk of micro-movements.

Conclusions

First, patients must understand the risks, benefits, and alternatives regarding single-tooth implant placement and timing. Same-day implants can only be used in specific situations, and patients need to be carefully evaluated for suitability.

Preplanning and experience from the implant surgeon, as well as thoroughly conducted care measures, are required for the success of this technique.

If you are not suitable for immediate dental implant placement, it is still worth considering delayed loading implants, even though treatment will take a little longer.

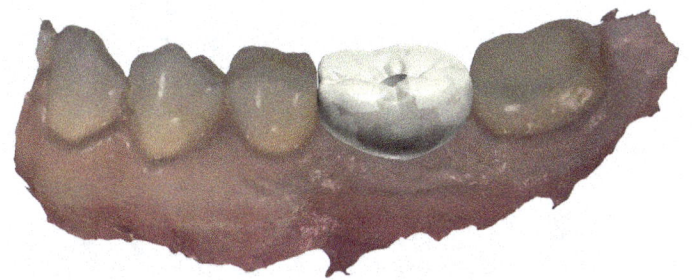

7. Prosthetic Phase

◆◆◆

The prosthetic phase begins once the implant is well integrated, or there is reasonable assurance that it will integrate.

Even in the event of early loading (when artificial teeth are attached to the implants in less than three months), many practitioners will place temporary teeth until osseointegration is confirmed.

The prosthetic phase of restoring an implant requires equal technical expertise as the surgical because of the biomechanical considerations, significantly when multiple teeth are restored.

The dentist will work to restore a functional bite (or occlusion), the aesthetics of the smile, and the structural integrity of the teeth to distribute the forces of the implants evenly.

Several steps are involved:

7.1 Removing The Temporary Restorations

All provisional restorations are removed. In some situations, the temporary restorations may be reused during the execution of the definitive prosthesis.

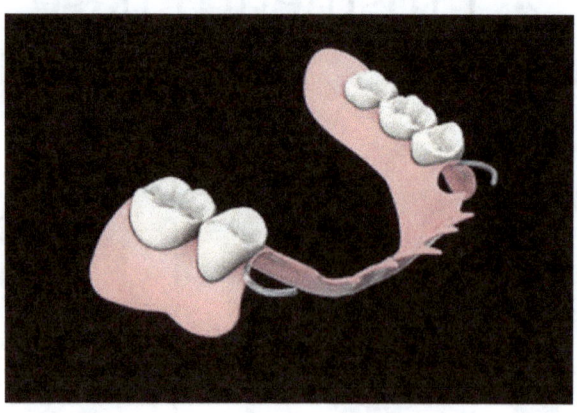

a temporary partial denture used to replace the missing teeth

7.2 Testing The Degree Of Osseointegration

When testing the level of osseointegration, certain factors need to be taken into account:

- the absence of pain
- clinical mobility around the implant fixture
- infection around the implants
- gingival bleeding

The *Periotest* is a specific device that measures the degree of implant mobility inside the bone. It has the advantage of measuring the levels of subclinical mobility using an ultrasonically vibrating probe.

The Periotest is successful in assessing the stability status of an implant. Still, it can detect the quantity of bony osseointegration only in terminal cases (3 to 6 months after the implant placement).

Therefore, it is advisable to combine this test with a dental radiography; radiography proved to be a more sensitive method of determining the degree of bone formation (or loss) around a dental implant.

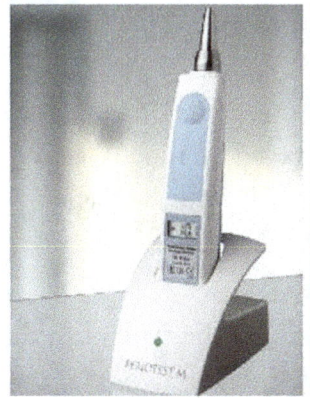

Periotest

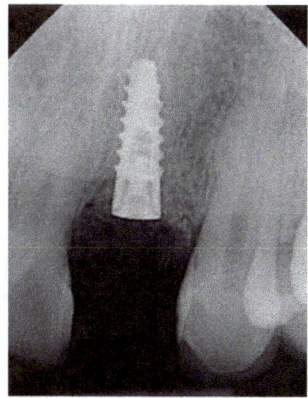

periapical radiography:
a well integrated dental implant

In conclusion, periapical radiographs, in addition to the Periotest device, were found to offer the most reliable assessment of an implant osseointegration status.

7.3 Removing The Healing Devices

The healing devices are specific devices screwed into the implant fixtures after the surgical placement. There are two possible options:

• **Healing abutment**

The healing abutment passes through the soft tissues and the surrounding gum tissue is adapted around it.

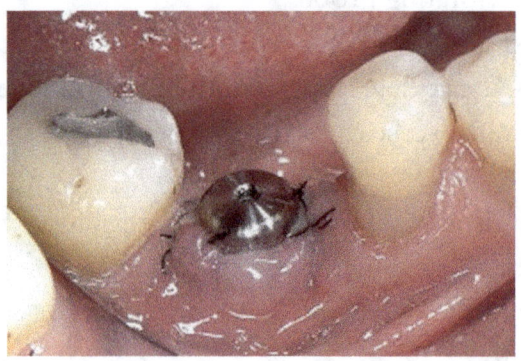

• **Cover screw**

The cover screw is flush with the surface of the dental implant and is designed to be entirely covered by mucosa. When a cover screw is used, the implant is "buried" and the tissue is closed to protect it completely.

Therefore, this procedure depends on the type of healing device that was used:

• If a *healing abutment* was used, simply unscrewing it with a specific key makes the removal.

• When a *cover screw* is positioned, a second procedure is needed to uncover the implant. The incision is very simple and painless.

7.4 Attaching The Implant Abutments

Implant abutments are artificial devices connected to the dental implants after the healing process. The abutments attach a crown, bridge, or removable denture to the implant fixtures.
There are two types of abutments:

• **Prefabricated abutments** - are the most common types and are usually delivered by manufacturing companies in a wide range of shapes and sizes along with the implants.

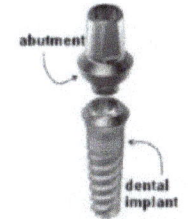

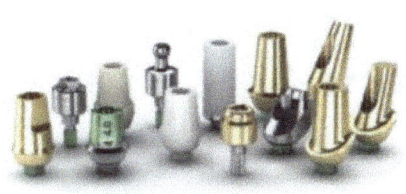

attaching the abutment to   *implant abutments*
the implant fixture   *of various types*

• **Custom-made abutments** are fabricated at the dental laboratory after an impression of the top of the implant is made with the adjacent teeth and gingiva.

Technique

The abutments are attached to the implant fixtures with a specific key regardless of the type.

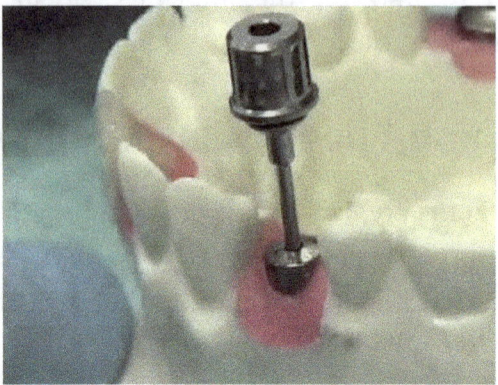

An abutment is not necessarily parallel to the long axis of the implant. Angulated abutments are utilized when the implant is at a different inclination in relation to the proposed prosthesis.

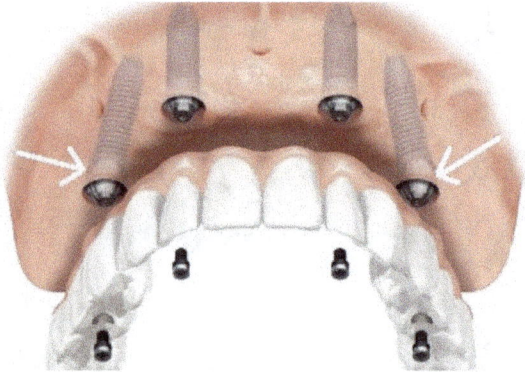

The primary purpose, in this case, is to make all artificial abutments parallel to each other.

7.5 The Dental Impression

A dental impression is an imprint of teeth, soft tissues, and surrounding oral structures. Dental impressions are used for a wide range of dental restorations and oral appliances (such as dental crowns and bridges, removable dentures, teeth whitening trays, and many more).

After the abutments are attached to the implants, your doctor will take an impression of all your teeth and send it to the dental lab where your designed restoration will be manufactured.

There are two ways your dentist may take the dental impressions:

a. Traditional impressions

Traditional impressions are formed with specific impression materials placed into plastic or metal trays. The trays are placed over your teeth until the dental impression material sets and hardens.

The dental impression forms an imprint (i.e., a 'negative' mould) of teeth and soft tissues, which the dental laboratory can then use to make a cast of the dentition.

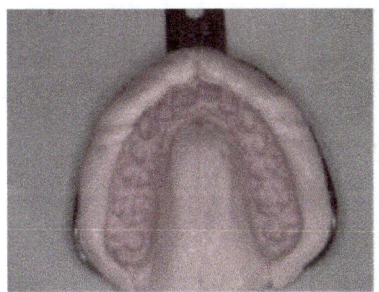
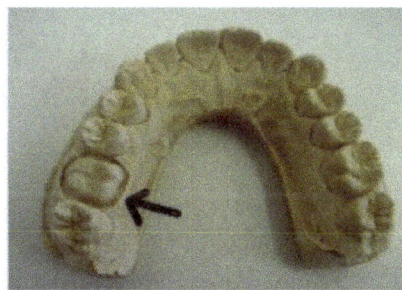

traditional dental impression   *dental cast*

b. Digital impressions

Digital impressions enable dentists to build a computer-generated, virtual replica of the teeth and soft tissues in the mouth.

During this procedure, the medical practitioner uses a digital scanner to capture thousands of pictures of your teeth and gums. The computer software will then combine the images together, creating a digital, 3D representation of the dental arches.

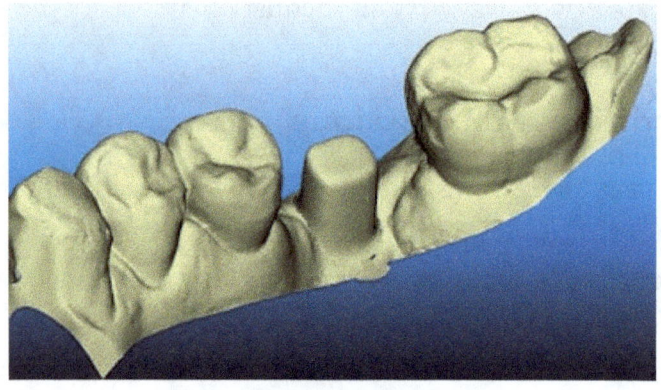

digital impression

The 3D representation will be electronically delivered to the dental lab.

In some variations, after the impression, the abutment is unscrewed from the implant and sent to the dental lab along with the impressions.

Bite registration

The bite registration shows the way the upper and lower teeth fit together. The long-term success of implants is determined, in part, by the forces they have to support. Therefore, restoring a proper occlusion (or bite) is one of the most important goals.

It is essential not to overload the implants with additional pressures and to distribute the chewing forces across all implant fixtures evenly.

The usual bite registration techniques often need to provide more data for the dental technician. In complex situations, especially when extensive restorations are designed, it is advisable to use advanced jaw tracking devices that provide additional details.

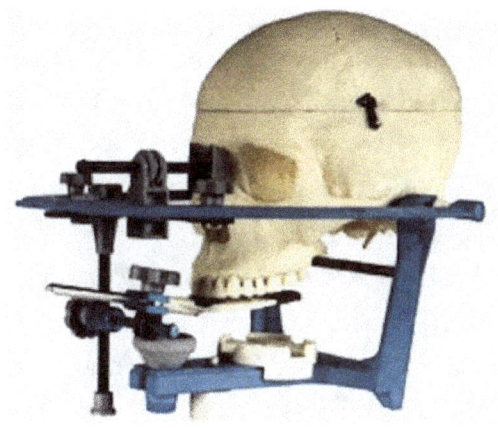

jaw tracking device

The jaw tracking devices provide details about the precise position of the maxilla and mandible against different anatomical structures of the head. This information is beneficial when manufacturing large restorations that must be highly accurate.

The bite registration can be digitally recorded if digital impression software is used.

All dental impressions, along with the bite registration and any other pertinent details for the dental technician, will be sent to the dental laboratory.

7.6 Dental Laboratory Stages

The dental lab is where the final restorations are constructed.

There are various ways of manufacturing a dental restoration, from traditionally fabricated reconstructions, where the dental technician manually builds up (layer by layer) the entire designed prosthesis to complete computer-designed and manufactured restorations.

a. Traditionally fabricated dental restorations

There are many ways a dental technician can manually construct dental restorations. Any prosthetic device, including dental crowns, bridges, or removable dentures, can be manually manufactured.

In subchapter 3.3.1: "*What Are Implant Supported Restorations Made Of?*" we discuss the various materials implant-supported prostheses can be made of as well as their main characteristics..

Generally, the dental technician will follow these steps:

• *Dental cast*

The dental cast is the positive reproduction of your teeth and surrounding tissues. To obtain the dental cast, the dental technician will pour a specific plaster inside the impression so it reaches all its details. All the designed restorations will be constructed on the dental cast.

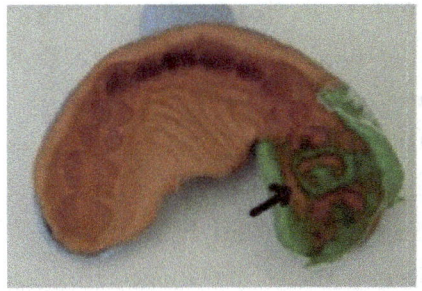

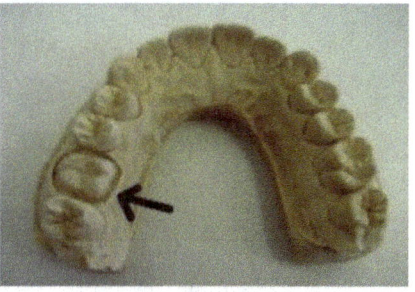

dental impression

*the dental cast obtained
from the impression*

• *Metal frame build-up*

Large bridges usually have a metal or zirconia frame that gives strength and durability to the entire restoration.

The aesthetic materials are then placed all around the supporting core so that no part of it remains visible.

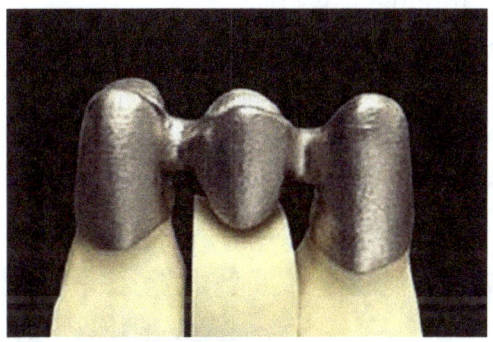

metal frame

Zirconia frames are computer-manufactured, but metal frames are often manually built. To do this, the dental technician will proceed as follows:

> • **Wax-Up**: the first step is to create the metal frame using a wax-up technique. The entire metal core is sculpted in wax at the precise shape and size, considering all aspects demanded by the particular clinical situation.

• **Investing** is the operation of surrounding the wax pattern with a material that can accurately duplicate its shape and anatomic features.

• **Casting The Metal Alloy**: where the wax pattern of the restoration is converted to a replicate in dental alloy.

• **Polishing And Finishing The Metal Frame**: even if all the steps were perfectly completed, minor touches are still required.

After the metal frame is completed, it is usually sent back to the dental practice for a fitting appointment.

• *Dental ceramics build-up*

Ceramics (also known as porcelain) will be placed all around the supporting core (either metal-base frame or zirconia frame) so that no part of it remains visible.

Dental ceramics have outstanding aesthetic features, giving the implant restoration an almost tooth-like appearance.

Porcelain is applied in multiple layers ranging from 4 to 7. Each layer has to be separately fired in special furnaces at high temperatures (up to 1000 degrees Celsius or 1830 Fahrenheit).

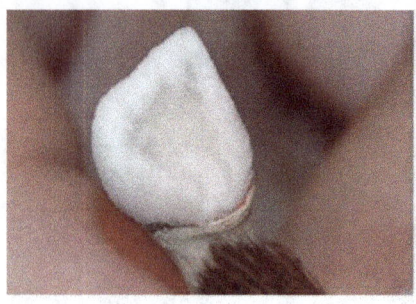
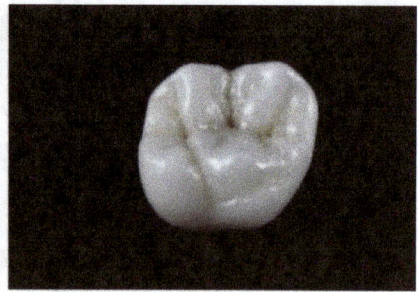

dental ceramics build-up   *a highly aesthetic dental ceramic crown*

The final layer, known as the glaze layer, gives the restoration a smooth surface and translucency that mimics tooth enamel.

b. Computer-designed and manufactured restorations

The CAD/CAM systems (Computer-Aided Design and Computer-Aided Manufacturing) are computerized systems used to design and manufacture various types of dental restorations.

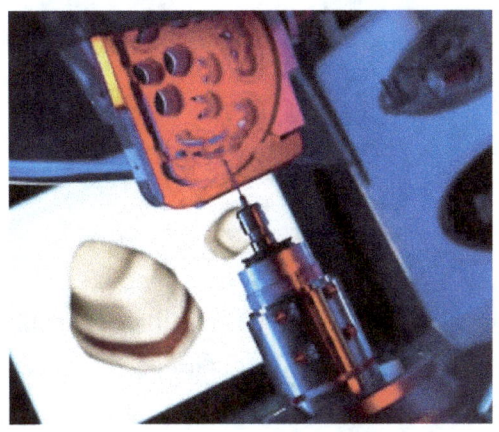

CAD/CAM system

Although CAD/CAM systems may be used to manufacture almost any type of reconstruction, implant dentistry generally uses them to construct all ceramics restorations and zirconia frames.

Process

- A prerequisite for computer-manufactured restorations is the digital impression.
- The digital impression draws the data into a computer. The main software creates the virtual restoration and sends the data to the *milling machine*.
- The milling machine is the part that fabricates the designed restoration by carving it out of a solid block of

zirconia or ceramic according to the information received from the computer.

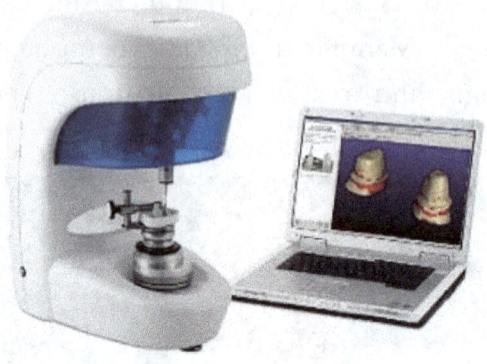

cad/cam system milling machine

• Zirconia frames are placed inside special furnaces at high temperatures (1500 degrees Celsius or 2730 Fahrenheit) for 6-7 hours, increasing the tensile strength of zirconia.

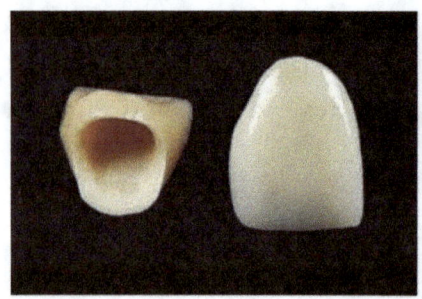
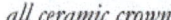
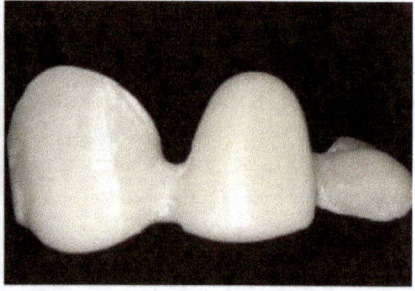

all ceramic crown   *zirconia frame*

Most of the time, zirconia frames will be manually layered with porcelain. Manually applied ceramics will give better aesthetic results because they possess a deep-set coloration due to the multi-layering.

c. Removable dentures

When a removable denture is designed, there is a slight difference in the manufacturing process. Usually, dentures are manually constructed at the dental lab.

Dentures are made of an acrylic base, a set of teeth, and special retainers. So, how does the dental technician manufacture the denture?

- First, the technician shapes and carves the wax on the dental cast; this is what the base of your finished dentures will look like.
- The technician will then set the teeth in the desired scheme, ensuring proper form and function. Generally, the teeth come in prefabricated sets of various sizes and are either acrylic or porcelain. Artificial teeth can also be custom-made at the dental lab.

The special retainers are also set up in the designed positions. After that, a fitting appointment at the dental practice is usually required.

- Finally, the technician injects acrylic into the base of the denture. Acrylic is injected to replace the wax and cured under pressure until the correct hardness is achieved.

Each denture is hand-finished using special burs and polished with polishing mops and paste to create a natural-looking luster.

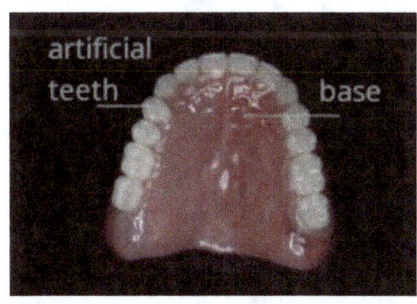 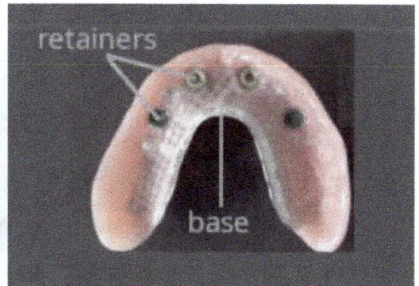

7.7 Fitting

One or more fitting appointments may be needed before the restoration is definitively attached to the dental implants. Your practitioner will check how well the prosthesis fits and make the necessary adjustments if the fitting is not perfect.

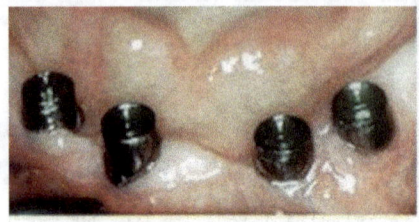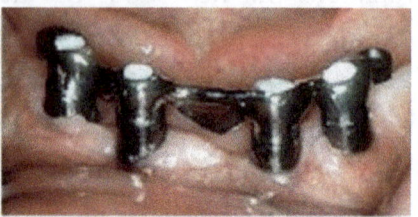

framework fitting for an implant supported denture

The bite adjustment

Any dental restoration must perfectly fit the patient's static and dynamic occlusion (or bite). This is a vital element, as a dysfunctional environment created by an inaccurately adjusted implant-supported restoration can lead to implant failure.

What is *static occlusion*?

> • **Static occlusion refers to contact between teeth when the jaw is closed and stationary.**

What is *dynamic occlusion*?

> • **Dynamic occlusion refers to occlusal contacts made when the jaw is moving. These contacts are made when the mandible moves sideways, forwards, backward, or at an angle.**

The patient closes the dental arches in the correct bite for the static occlusion while the dynamic occlusion is checked during various mandible movements.

The articulating paper is the tool used to highlight occlusal contacts by marking areas on teeth or restorations where contacts are made during biting or other jaw movements.

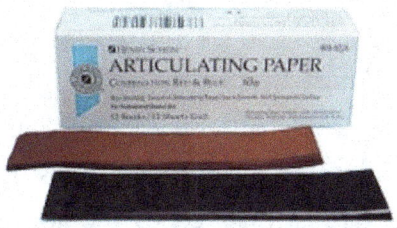

articulating paper

The bite adjustment procedure is done by placing a strip of articulating paper between the teeth while the desired mandibular movements are performed. The areas where restorations need occlusal adjustments appear as colored points or lines.

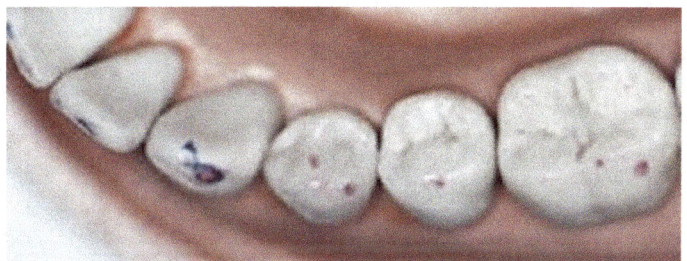

Adjustments are made with diamond or tungsten carbide burs, and the bite is rechecked until the reconstruction fits perfectly.

When the fitting is perfect, the implant prosthesis can be definitively attached to the implants.

7.8 Attaching The Prosthesis

How the implant restoration attaches to the implants depends on the type of prosthesis designed.

a. Fixed prosthesis

A fixed prosthesis is when a person cannot remove the denture or teeth from their mouth. Where the prosthetic is fixed, the dental crown or bridge is attached to the abutment with either lag screws or cement.

• *The prosthesis is attached with lag screws*

The restoration is secured with screws that traverse the dental crowns and attach to the threaded holes inside the abutments. After the screws are positioned, the holes that penetrate the crowns are sealed with a composite material.

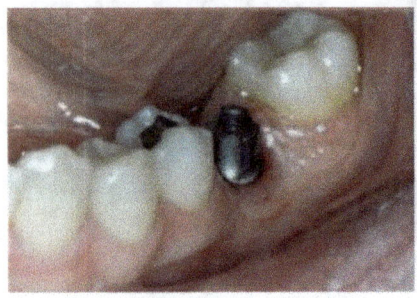 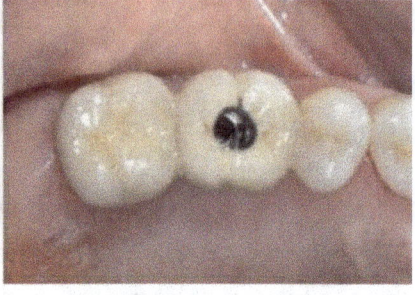

artificial abutment with a threaded hole   *the crown is secured with a lag-screw*

Another variation is when the crown and abutment are one piece, and the lag screw traverses both to secure the one-piece structure to the internal thread on the implant.

• *The prosthesis is secured with dental cement*

In this case, the restoration is secured with dental cement, just like crowns and bridges are attached to natural teeth.

Dental cement is a specific material used to secure definitive restorations (such as crowns or bridges) to abutment teeth or dental implants. They are hard, brittle materials formed by mixing powder and liquid together.

Dental cements develop a strong bond with the restoration, have a high biocompatibility, and provide good marginal sealing to prevent marginal leakage and protect the dental tissues from external stimuli.

Cementation technique

• The dental cement is prepared by mixing the powder and liquid according to the manufacturer's instructions.

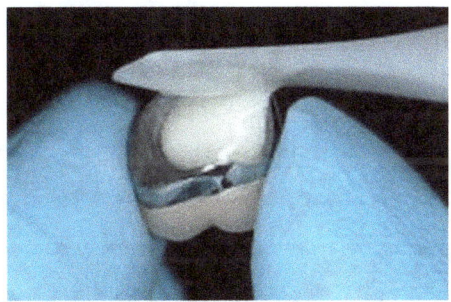

• When the cement reaches optimum consistency (a "creamy" consistency), it is placed inside the crowns carefully to cover all interior walls.

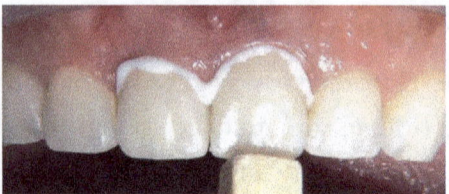

• The restoration is positioned on the abutment, applying gentle pressure until it reaches the final position.

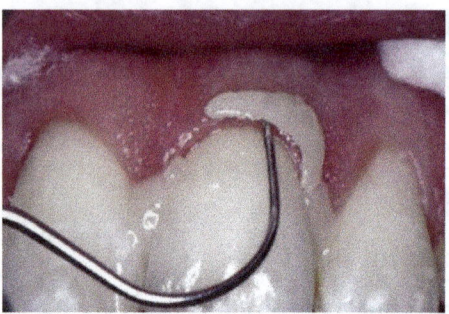

• After the primary setting, the excess cement is removed with a dental explorer.

b. Removable dentures

Removable dentures are held in place by special adapters (or retainers). Generally, a male-adapter is connected to the implant, and a female-adapter is housed in the denture.

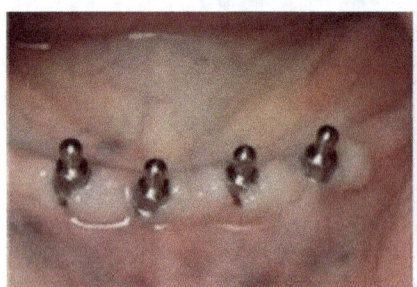

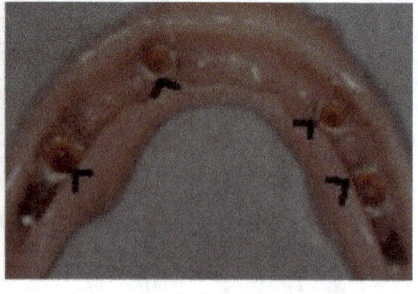

*the male-adapters
are attached to the implants*

*the female-adapters
are housed in the denture*

The retainers allow movement of the denture but enough retention to improve the quality of life for denture wearers compared to conventional dentures.

Removable dentures should be removed daily to clean the denture and gum area.

After the restoration is permanently attached to the implants, your doctor will schedule one or more appointments for periodic monitoring.

Immediate care:

- protect the part with the restoration in the early days
- thorough oral hygiene
- report any discomfort

7.9 Immediate Follow-Up

After the prosthesis is definitively attached to the implants, it takes a little time for the dental tissues to adapt to the new situation. Therefore, some minor reactions may occur.

Most often, the symptoms gradually disappear after a short period or after simple interventions performed at the dental office.

• Light pain in the gums

In many cases, the practitioner will try to hide the margin of the restoration. The line is unsightly to be exposed, so the dentist would like to place the margin below the gum line.

As a result, you may feel mild pain in the gums until the soft tissues adapt to the new situation. Usually, the pain goes away after several days without any medication (although your clinician may prescribe some mild pain relievers).

• Pain or discomfort when chewing

If you experience pain or discomfort when biting down on something, the bite needs to be readjusted.

In these cases, it is imperative to contact your dentist. It is essential that the prosthesis perfectly fits in the bite so all chewing forces are evenly distributed on the implants.

• Removable dentures

New removable dentures or overdentures may feel awkward for a few weeks until the body becomes accustomed to them. Dentures are generally larger than fixed restorations (crowns, bridges), so the dental tissues need time to adapt.

It is not unusual to experience minor irritation or soreness in the early days. When small lesions appear on the mucosa (see the image on the next page), the removable denture needs minor adjustments performed at the dental office.

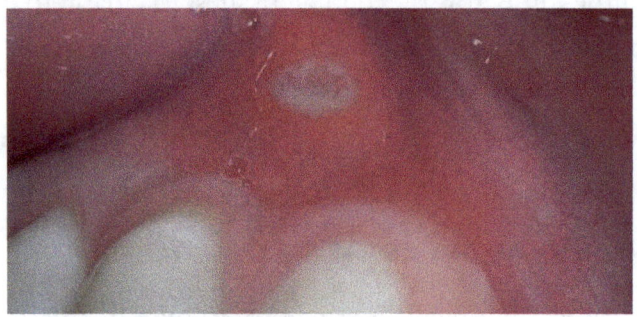

*small lesions caused by a
recently manufactured removable denture*

The saliva flow may temporarily increase. As the mouth becomes accustomed to the dentures, these problems should go away.

Follow-up appointments with the dentist are generally needed after a denture is inserted so the fit can be checked and adjusted. If any problem persists, particularly irritation or soreness, be sure to inform your doctor.

Generally, it takes time to get used to any new restoration. However, after the accommodation period, the implant-supported prosthesis should look, function, and feel like regular teeth after some time.

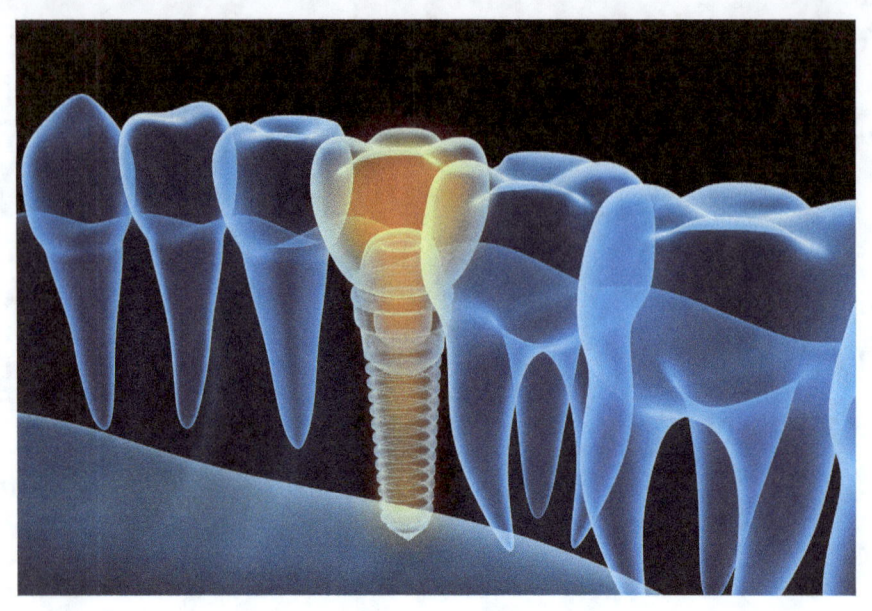

8. Dental Implants. Care And Risks

❖❖❖

8.1 Dental Implants. Care And Maintenance

Dental implants require regular professional maintenance as well as proper home care. Taking good care of dental implants is vital for long-term success.

• Oral hygiene

Proper and thorough oral hygiene is a prerequisite for successful dental implant rehabilitation. Poor oral hygiene dramatically increases the risk of failure.

After placement, implants need to be cleaned with a Teflon instrument (or the type your doctor recommends) to remove plaque. Because of the more precarious blood supply to the gingiva, care should be taken with dental floss.

You should carefully clean fixed implant restorations (crowns, bridges) as well. For example, a bridge should be brushed at least twice daily with fluoride paste and cleaned between the teeth and under the bridge with dental floss, interdental cleaners, and water jets.

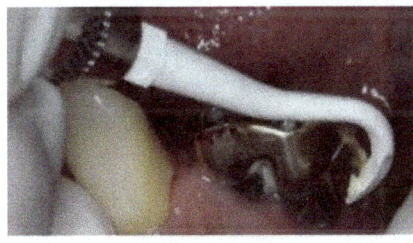

dental implant cleaned with a Teflon instrument

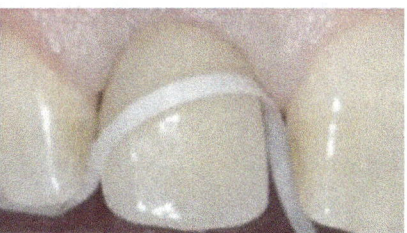

implant supported crown: flossing

Removable dentures supported by implants should be removed daily and cleaned separately. Particular attention should be given to the underneath gum area.

• Periodic monitoring

Regular checkups should be conducted at least twice a year. During checkups, the practitioner assesses the overall situation, verifies implant stability and integration, the status of the prosthetic devices, and makes the necessary adjustments.

The oral mucosa is checked, and professional teeth cleaning and tartar scaling are performed. You should report any pain, discomfort, or unusual signs during the checkups.

• Implant restorations should not be overloaded

It is advisable to avoid biting on hard pieces of food: peanuts or pistachios, very hard bread crumbs, etc.

Moreover, some conditions can harm dental implants and prosthetic devices. For example, bruxism is a condition that involves involuntary habitual grinding of the teeth, typically during sleep.

It would be best to inform your doctor as soon as you notice the first signs of such conditions.

• Maintenance of removable dentures

Removable dentures and overdentures require continuous maintenance. The female adapters housed in the denture need to be changed or refreshed every one to two years because they wear off. The operation is straightforward and quick.

Relining

Relining or rebasing is indicated when a removable denture fit has worsened, resulting in an unstable denture or tissue trauma. A denture relining involves refitting the tissue side of the denture to custom fit the mouth.

A removable denture fit can worsen due to 2 possible causes:

- The manufacturing material (usually acrylic) from the base of the denture has worn of
  - The bone beneath the denture underwent a process of remodeling and has diminished its height.

Relining involves replacing the fitting surface with a new material, usually cold or heat-cured acrylic or tissue conditioner.

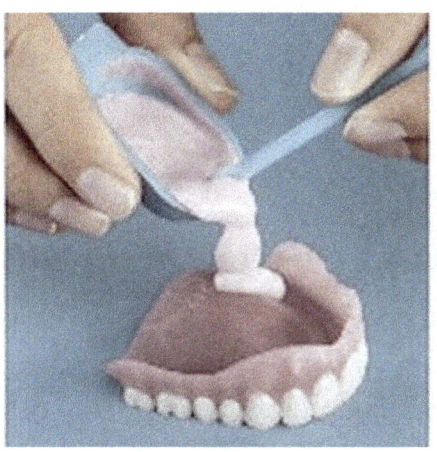

removable denture relining

Relining can be carried out directly (at the dental office) or, more often, indirectly (at the dental lab). Generally, up to one appointment is required, and the procedure is not very expensive.

For example, if the relining is done at the dental office, the dentist will apply the soft or hard relining resin to the dentures. He will then place the dentures back in your mouth, and you should bite down gently to make an impression in the resin. Once the resin hardens, the reline is complete.

8.2 Dental Implants. Risks And Complications

Even though enormous technical advances have significantly improved the quality of dental treatments, accidents and complications may still occur, and it is vital to be aware of this.

The placement of dental implants is a surgical procedure and carries the usual risks of surgery. Other complications may occur in the first 6 months after the placement and even in the long-term.

1. Risks and complications during implant surgery

Placement of dental implants is a surgical procedure and carries the usual risks of surgery. If additional surgical procedures are performed (sinus lift, bone graft, etc.), they also have the normal risks.

However, the risk of complications is considered to be very low - less than 5 percent, according to current statistics. Problems are rare, and when they do occur, they are usually minor and easily treated.

• Bleeding

Life-threatening events associated with dental implants are extremely rare, but some severe bleeding may occur, especially if large blood vessels are injured during surgery.

If such an accident should occur, treatment includes compression, vasoconstrictive medication, cautery, or ligation of arteries. Most of the time, bleeding is kept under control.

• Infection

Infection from bacteria is a common risk to any surgery. In modern days, less than 1% of surgeries result in an infection, and most of those infections are minor.

An infection at the implant site during surgery or in the early days after surgery can increase the risk of implant failure. Pre-op antibiotics reduce the risk of implant failure but have little impact on the risk of infection.

Proper oral hygiene after surgery is essential. A clean mouth will heal faster, and the risk of infection is reduced if the mouth is not riddled with bacteria and food debris.

• Nerve damage

The most common issue is when the inferior alveolar nerve (located inside the mandible) is accidentally damaged during surgery. After surgery, patients may experience lingering pain, tingling, and numbness in the teeth, gums, lips (mainly the lower lip), or chin for an undetermined time.

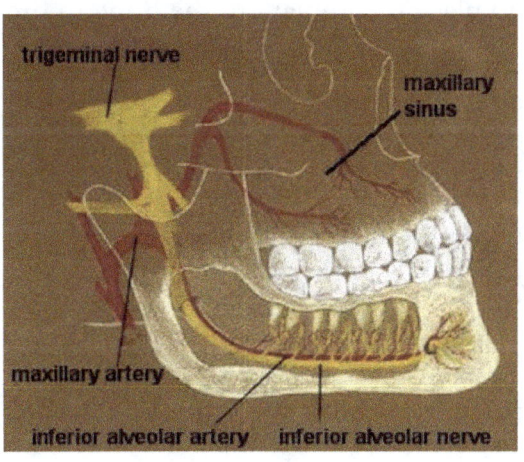

important anatomical structures
that can be damaged during implant surgery

If the nerve damage is minor, patients will likely recover.

• Sinus problems

Sinus problems occur when dental implants placed in the upper jaw protrude into one of the sinus cavities. Careful planning and precise surgery execution are essential to avoid this accident.

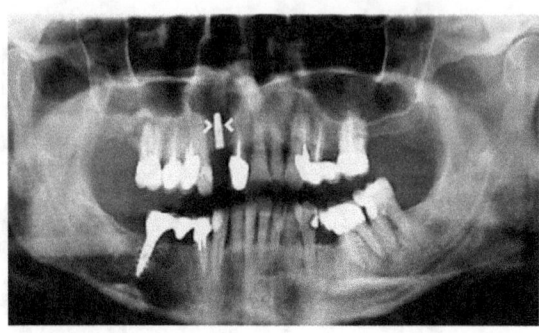

panoramic film: a dental implant protrudes into the sinus cavity

Even if sinus complications do not occur in every case, these implants have a high risk of failure because of insufficient bone support.

• Lack of stability

An inability to place the implant in the bone to provide stability (referred to as *primary stability*) increases the risk of failure to osseointegration.

Some research even suggests that the primary stability of the implant in bone is a more critical determinant of the success of implant integration rather than a certain period of healing time.

• Other risks

Other accidents may occur during the surgical placement; these are extremely rare: damage (and possible devitalization) of adjacent teeth or other surrounding structures, necrosis of the flap of tissue around the implant, or mandibular fracture.

2. Risks and complications in the first 6 months

These complications occur in the first 6 months after implant placement. The most common complication is the failure to integrate.

• *Failure to integrate*

An implant failure to integrate in the first 6 months can first be related to some general or local factors:

> • general conditions such as uncontrolled diabetes, untreated osteoporosis, radiation exposure on the head and neck, or other severe conditions
> • improper oral hygiene
> • heavy smokers or high alcohol consumption
> • various accidents during surgery: infection, puncture of a sinus cavity, etc

However, the latest research suggests that primary implant stability is the principal factor.

For this, an implant needs to be surrounded by a healthy quantity of bone, and it has to be placed in the bone to provide stability for the implant. Loosening implant posts have a higher risk of failure.

An implant is tested between 8 and 24 weeks to determine bone integration. The clinical signs to determine implant success are the absence of pain, mobility, infection, and gingival bleeding.

The osseointegration status is then tested on radiographs and with specific devices (e.g., Periotest).

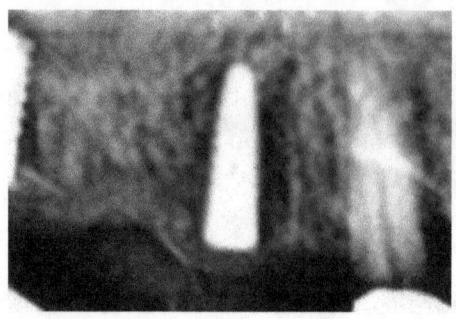

dental X-ray: implant failure to integrate; it is considered that a radiographic lucency greater than 1.5 mm around a dental implant is a sign of failure

What is *Radiographic Lucency?*

 • In radiology, lucency is a darker region normally caused by soft tissues, air, or liquid.

It is the opposite of opacity, which has a whiter shade and is caused by hard tissues (teeth, bone), metal, or artifacts.

Lucency around a dental implant signifies *bone loss.*

While there is significant variation in the rate at which implants fail to integrate (due to individual risk factors), the approximate values are **1 to 6 percent**.

3. Long term complications

Long-term implant failures may be caused by an improper design of the prosthetic restoration or by inappropriate care and maintenance. Regardless of the cause, implants fail due to either loss of bone around them or a mechanical failure of the implant.

There are also the risks associated with the prosthetic components, which, over time, can wear off, chip, break, or cause a lack of satisfaction on the part of the patient.

• *Peri-implantitis*

Peri-implantitis is a destructive inflammatory process affecting the soft and hard tissues surrounding an osseointegrated implant in function. Peri-implantitis is an infectious disease; various factors can cause this condition:

- improper oral hygiene
- excessive mechanical load on the implant
- the status of the tissue surrounding the implant
- patients with diabetes
- heavy smokers

Diagnosis is based on changes of color in the gingiva, bleeding, and probing depth of peri-implant pockets and suppuration. The X-ray shows a gradual loss of bone height around the implant.

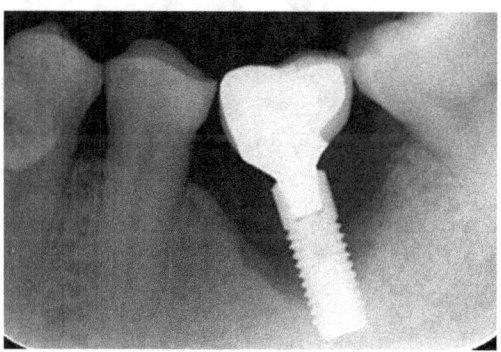

peri-implantitis

If peri-implantitis is diagnosed, treatment will depend on the amount of bone loss and the aesthetic impact of the implant in question.

The therapeutic approach can range from local debridements around the implant fixture, antibiotics, antiseptics, and ultrasonic and laser treatments to regenerative procedures using a bone graft.

• *Fracture of the implant*

The fracture is a mechanical failure of the implant. Fractures may occur when implants are too short or too thin. The implant can fracture at various levels :

> • The fracture of the implant and abutment screw is a catastrophic failure, and usually, the fixture and the prosthetic components cannot be salvaged (image a).
> • When only the abutment fractures, the abutment and the crown would need replacement, but the implant fixture can sometimes be salvaged (image b).

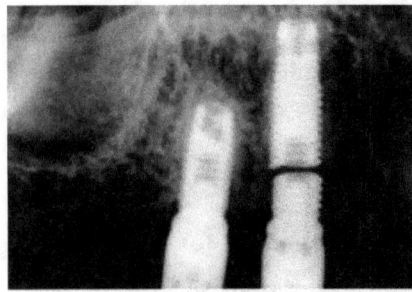
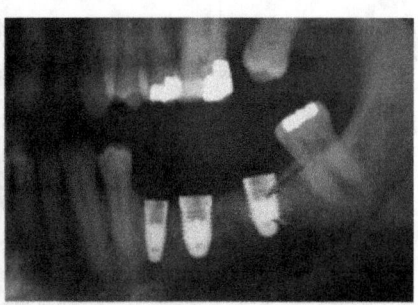

a : fracture of the implant   *b : fracture of the abutment screws*

• *Gingival recession*

The most common cause of gingival recession is gingivitis, an inflammatory disease of the gums mainly caused by improper oral hygiene.

Recession of the gingiva leads to exposure of the metal abutment under a dental crown. In other situations, black triangles caused by bone loss and the retraction of the papilla appear between implants and natural teeth.

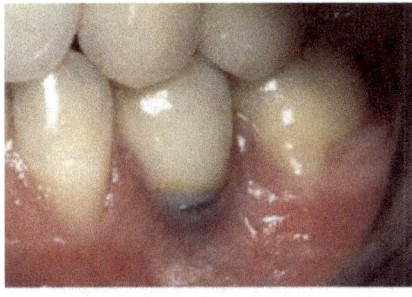
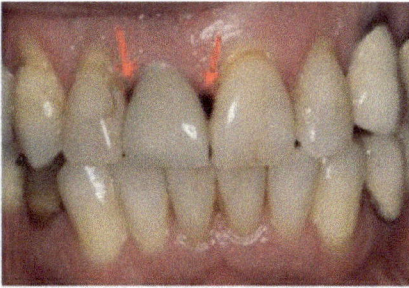

gingival recession   *black triangles*

Some of these conditions may be improved with a *soft tissue graft*. Before any surgery, all causative agents have to be removed.

• *Prosthetic restoration risks*

Besides the implants, there are risks associated with the prosthetic components.

First, poor aesthetics, including a high smile line, poor gingival quality, and missing papillae, plus the difficulty in matching th form and shade of natural teeth, may lead to a lack of satisfaction on the part of the patient (assuming the patient does not have unrealistic expectations).

Over time, prostheses can wear off, chip, break, detach, change aesthetic appearance, or suffer other complications.

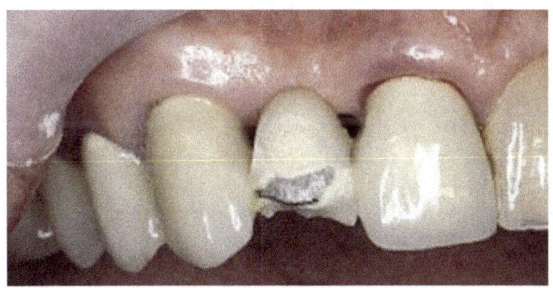

chipped porcelain restoration

Most of the time, the implant fixtures last longer than the prosthesis. The lifespan for a prosthetic reconstruction is around 15 years, while a well-positioned implant fixture can last a lifetime.

Additionally, removable dentures and overdentures need regular maintenance.

Patients who wear implant-supported prostheses should ideally be free of pain or any other unpleasant signs, able to chew and taste, and pleased with the aesthetics.

Implants should be tested at least twice a year during regular checkups. Criteria for the success are:
- the absence of pain
- the absence of mobility
- no radiographic lucency greater than 1.5 mm around implants
- the lack of suppuration or bleeding in the soft tissues
- adequate function and aesthetics in the prosthetic

8.3 Dental Implants Failure: Possible Reasons

Dental implants are considered today as the best treatment option for tooth loss. The great advantage of a dental implant is that it replaces the missing tooth in the most natural way possible.

Implant-supported restorations give great aesthetic results and can last longer than most other treatment options, like traditional dental bridges or removable dentures.

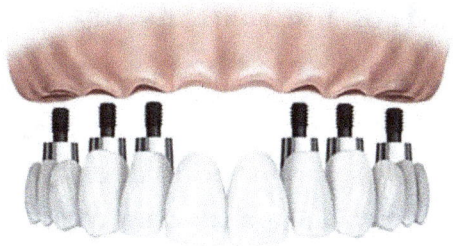

However, no treatment option gives one hundred percent positive results when dealing with the human body. That is why dental implant failure is a fact that should be accepted.

The average success rate of dental implants is around 95%. It means that if a dentist places 500 implants, an average of 25 of those will fail.

Even if there are many reasons for implant failure, the most common cause of failure is when the patient and the dentist try to settle for cheaper solutions. Dental implant treatments are not cheap, and there is a good reason for that.

Next, we will summarize the most common reasons for dental implant failure:

• Inadequate planning

Planning for dental implants is the most critical step of the entire treatment. Besides a thorough examination, dental implants need specific imaging methods such as panoramic X-rays or computed tomography, especially in more complex cases.

Modern computer software is also available; this can be viable in assessing dental implant position and placement. Some dentists may try to shortcut these tests or go for cheaper solutions; this can increase the rate of implant failure.

• Inadequate information about the patient's general health or medical history

Some severe general conditions make anesthesia, surgical procedures, and the overall placement inadvisable. At the same time, other situations should be evaluated on a case-by-case basis and may require some preliminary treatments.

A thorough interview and diagnosis should be done to avoid complications later on.

• Improper planning or execution of adjunctive surgical procedures

For an implant to osseointegrate, it needs to be surrounded by a healthy quantity of bone. Therefore, the bone will have to achieve an adequate width and height. Implants placed in inadequate bone have a higher risk of failure.

The adjunctive surgical procedures are planned to increase the bone amount or reposition anatomical structures that might interfere with the implants (such as the maxillary sinus or the alveolar nerve).

Some clinical situations will not require adjunctive procedures. However, when the case calls, they are essential for long-term success.

• Inadequate dental implant fixtures

Even though hundreds of companies manufacture dental implant fixtures, only a few have really been keen on their research programs. Dental implants must undergo extreme research, and research programs are expensive.

This is one of the reasons implant procedures are expensive: because the dentist uses high-quality fixtures.

• Implant surgery risks

Placement of dental implants is a surgical procedure and carries the normal risks of surgery. Some of these risks may lead to an increase in the rate of failure.

For example, the inability to place the implant in the bone to provide stability (the primary stability of the implant) increases the risk of failure to osseointegration. Modern imaging methods (such as CT scans or CBCT) can significantly reduce these risks.

• Restoring an improper occlusion or bite

The long-term success of implants is determined, in part, by the forces they have to support. Therefore, restoring a proper occlusion (or bite) is one of the most important goals.

It is essential not to overload the implants with additional pressures and to distribute the chewing forces of the implants evenly. Otherwise, there is a high risk of failure.

• Inadequate care

Dental implants require regular professional maintenance as well as proper home care. Taking good care of dental implants is vital for long-term success.

What can we do to avoid problems with dental implants?

Try to find an experienced doctor you'll trust; you can talk to former patients to ask for their feedback, or a friend or relative can recommend a dental surgeon.

Do not opt for cheap solutions; if your dentist recommends modern imaging methods or adjunctive surgery, take his advice;

remember, it will cost you much more if the implants fail in a short time.

Follow all the care measures, and remember that regular checkups should be conducted at least twice a year.

References

American Academy of Implant Dentistry: What are dental implants?
https://aaid-implant.org/faqs/what-are-dental-implants/

American Academy of Implant Dentistry: Dental Implants,
Alternative Techniques

American Academy of Periodontology: Multiple Tooth Implants
https://www.perio.org/for-patients/periodontal-treatments-and-procedures/dental-implant-procedures/multiple-tooth-dental-implants/

WebMD: Dental Implants
https://www.webmd.com/oral-health/dental-implants#1

Wikipedia: Dental Implant
https://en.wikipedia.org/wiki/Dental_implant

American Dental Association: Implants

Dear Doctor, A Patient Education Company: Same-Day Tooth
Replacement With Dental Implants

The National Center for Biotechnology Information: Role of primary
stability for successful osseointegration of dental implants: Factors of
influence and evaluation
https://www.ncbi.nlm.nih.gov/pmc/articles/PMC3873594/

Your Dentistry Guide: Implants vs Bridges
https://www.yourdentistryguide.com/implants-vs-bridges/

Carefree Dental: Dental Implants vs Bridges: How to Know What's
Best for You, Written by: Carefree Dental

Pierre Simonis, Thomas Dufour, Henri Tenenbaum: Long-term
implant survival and success: a 10-16-year follow-up of non-submerged dental implants

Liu, Chia-Hui; Lin, Cheng-Jyun; Hu, Ya-Han; You, Zi-Hung:
Predicting the Failure of Dental Implants Using Supervised Learning
Techniques

Misch CE: Contemporary Implant Dentistry

R. Palmer, Paul J. Palmer, Leslie C. Howe, British Dental Association: A clinical guide to implants in dentistry

Jacques Malet, Francis Mora, Philippe Bouchard: Implant dentistry at a glance

Norbert Cionca, Dena Hashim, Andrea Mombelli: Zirconia dental implants: where are we now, and where are we heading?

Spector L: Computer-aided dental implant planning

Marco Esposito, Maria Gabriella Grusovin, Ilias p Polyzos, Pietro Felice, Helen V Worthington: Timing of implant placement after tooth extraction: immediate, immediate-delayed or delayed implants? A Cochrane systematic review

Marco Esposito, Maria Gabriella Grusovin, Yun Shane Chew, Paul Coulthard, Helen V Worthington: One-stage versus two-stage implant placement. A Cochrane systematic review of randomised controlled clinical trials

Sclar A: Soft tissue and esthetic considerations in implant dentistry

Marco Esposito, Maria Gabriella Grusovin, Hassan Maghaireh, Helen V Worthington: Interventions for replacing missing teeth: different times for loading dental implants

Momen A Atieh, Ahmad H Atieh, Alan G T Payne, Warwick J Duncan: Immediate loading with single implant crowns: a systematic review and meta-analysis

Wirley Goncalves Assunção, Valentim Adelino Ricardo Barao, Juliana Aparecida Delben, Érica Alves Gomes, Lucas Fernando Tabata: A comparison of patient satisfaction between treatment with conventional complete dentures and overdentures in the elderly: a literature review

Wingrove S: Focus on implant home care Before, during, and after restoration

Yanfei Zhu, Xinyi Zheng, Guanqi Zeng, Yi Xu, Xinhua Qu, Min Zhu, and Eryi Luc: Clinical efficacy of early loading versus conventional loading of dental implants

Papaspyridakos P, Chen CJ, Singh M, Weber HP, Gallucci GO: Success criteria in implant dentistry: a systematic review

Fawad Javed, George E. Romanos: The role of primary stability for successful immediate loading of dental implants. A literature reviewGoodacre CJ, Bernal G, Rungcharassaeng K, Kan JY: Clinical complications with implants and implant prostheses

Esposito M, Ardebili Y, Worthington HV: Interventions for replacing missing teeth: different types of dental implants

Jokstad A: Osseointegration and Dental Implants

Lindhe J, Lang NP, Karring T: Clinical Periodontology and Implant Dentistry 5th edition

Indications of implants. http://alentinogroup.com/robert-half-zgloxlu/754d4e-indications-of-implants

Dental Implants – Dr. Pillai's Sacred Heart Dental Clinic in Mumbai. https://www.drpillai.in/dental-implants/

https://www.crownsnow.com/dental-implants-help-restore-confidence-in-your-smile/

Dental Implant Vs Crown - Dental News Network. https://sandiegoinvisaligndentist.org/dental-implant-vs-crown/

Abutment (dentistry) - Wikipedia. https://en.wikipedia.org/wiki/Abutment_(dentistry)

Assal, P. "The Osseointegration of Zirconia Dental Implants." PubMed, 2013, https://pubmed.ncbi.nlm.nih.gov/23965893

Dental Zircon – Lorans. https://www.loransmedical.com/dental-veneers-2/

CT Scan - Periodontal & Implant Excellence. https://perio-implantpb.com/services/CT-Scan/

Sinus lift - Wikipedia. https://en.wikipedia.org/wiki/Sinus_lift

Osseointegration And Dental Implants - Implants Pro Center. https://www.implantsprocentersanfrancisco.com/osseointegration-and-dental-implants/

Same Day Dental Implants & Immediate Loading. https://www.dentalimplantcostguide.com/same-day-immediate-loading/

All-On-4 Dental Implants cost - Cost | Payment Options | Financing. https://www.drarocha.com/all-on-4-dental-implants-cost.html

Dental Implant Failure - Possible Reasons | Dental Treatment Guide. https://www.dental-treatment-guide.com/dental-implants/dental-implant-failure-possible-reasons

About The Author

George Ghidrai MD

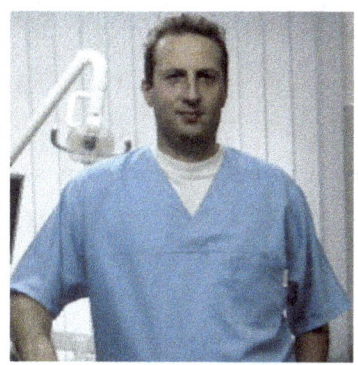

George Ghidrai, MD, is a General Dental Practitioner with over 20 years of experience. As a dental practitioner, Dr. Ghidrai has been actively treating patients at three dental clinics over the past 20 years.

Dr. Ghidrai's primary areas of expertise include cosmetic dentistry, tooth restoration, and prosthetic dentistry. In addition to being involved in direct patient care, he has also devoted much of his time to patient education. In 2013, he created *Infodentis.com*, a website that provides patients with extensive information on various dental procedures and mouth conditions.

Expertise

- Prosthetic and Implant Dentistry
- General Dentistry
- Teeth Whitening and Cosmetic Dentistry
- Content Writing

Education

Dr. George Ghidrai obtained his bachelor's degree in dentistry from the University of Medicine and Pharmacy "Iuliu Hatieganu" Cluj-Napoca, Romania. He then received his MD specializing in "General Dentistry" at the same University in 2003.

He worked for three different dental clinics, spending time on a variety of clinical cases. At present, he owns a Dental Practice in his hometown, Clu-Napoca.

Experience

Besides his clinical experience, Dr. Ghidrai has been actively involved in developing and creating patient-education content on the platform *Infodentis.com* as well as for other websites and publications.